Guide to Pulmonary Fibrosis &

Interstitial Lung Diseases

Written by

Noah Greenspan, PT, DPT, CCS, EMT-B

with **PF/ILD Patients:**

Charlene Marshall, BaSC, MA

(Facilitator)

Linda Gorman

René Hakkenberg

Thomas Hoks

Ann Kelley

John LaJeunesse

Grace McKeown

Ruth O'Bryan

Don Prager

Ronald Reid

Edited by Noah Greenspan, PT, DPT, CCS, EMT-B

Foreword by Robert Kaner, MD

Guide to Pulmonary Fibrosis & Interstitial Lung Diseases

Noah Greenspan, PT, DPT, CCS, EMT-B

Pulmonary Wellness Foundation
6 East 39th Street, NYC 10016
Suite 400
Telephone: 212.921.0214

www.pulmonarywellness.org
noah@pulmonarywellness.org

This project was made possible
by an Anonymous donation
in Honor of John and Lauren Veronis

If you find this book helpful, won't you please consider
supporting the Pulmonary Wellness Foundation's
mission to provide free educational opportunities
and experiences for people living with respiratory
disease through your tax-deductible donation at:

www.pulmonarywellness.org/thank-you/.

Contents

In Memoriam

The initial concept for this book was developed in collaboration with a very special friend, not just to me, but to very many in the pulmonary fibrosis community. Kim Fredrickson was a Licensed Marriage and Family Therapist, writer, journalist, advocate, *and IPF patient*. The last time I saw Kim, she was in the hospital, waiting for a lung transplant at the University of California San Francisco Medical Center. We had agreed to do a book that would be a hybrid between her book, *Pulmonary Fibrosis Journey: A Counselor and Fellow Patient Walks With You*, and mine, *Ultimate Pulmonary Wellness*. Unfortunately, shortly after we had begun this process, our greatest fear was realized. Kim passed away before she got her transplant and before we could complete the book. But the fire was already lit, and I promised her that in the event of her death, I would somehow bring our book to fruition. I hope she likes it.

I also want to recognize and thank another one of my patients, Sylvia Johnson. Sylvia also had IPF and was one of the few individuals who literally did *everything* necessary to live her best life. Sylvia was a Brooklyn girl, so you already know she was tough, but to show you just how tough she was, Sylvia used to travel from what we Brooklynites affectionately refer to as "the BK" to our Center in Manhattan, pushing a cart with 12 E tanks of oxygen and a non-rebreather mask. One of the best days of my life was when Sylvia, her daughter, Aisha, Francesca Harrison, my dog, *Monkey*, and I walked around Central Park in the blazing hot summer sun, taking turns pushing that cart.

We also wish to acknowledge three very special friends and co-authors of this book, who started this journey with us, but who sadly passed away before our work was completed. Ann Kelley, Thomas Hoks, and my buddy Don Prager, aka Donnie Vapor; your presence was felt throughout, and you are dearly missed.

Noah Greenspan

"The Prayer" by Don Prager aka Donnie Vapor

♪ *Got the news the other day* ♪ ♪ *Three to five I'm going away* ♪ ♪ *And it shook me to the bones* ♪ ♪ *Never felt so more alone* ♪ ♪ *I just want to blink my eyes and be okay* ♪ ♪ *We live our lives in passing days* ♪ ♪ *Might have strolled at rat race pace* ♪ ♪ *One day it punched me in the nose* ♪ ♪ *Suddenly my aura froze* ♪ ♪ *Oh my God there's gotta be another way* ♪ ♪ *And there is* ♪ ♪ *Smile every day at each other* ♪ ♪ *Let them know you care* ♪ ♪ *Awake every day and discover magic in the air* ♪ ♪ *Spreading love and inspiration* ♪ ♪ *Well that would be my prayer* ♪ ♪

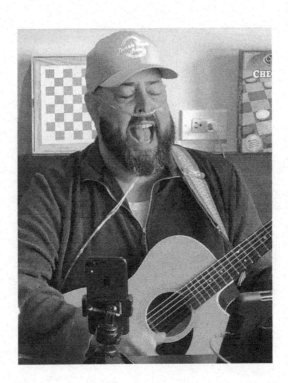

Foreword by Robert J. Kaner, MD

Patient-reported outcomes, such as shortness of breath and chronic cough, are key metrics in understanding how interstitial lung disease affects people's lives. Armed with this new perspective, we have come to understand the very substantial physical and psychological benefits of pulmonary rehabilitation for individuals living with moderate to advanced interstitial lung disease (ILD) of all types. Dr. Noah Greenspan has been a visionary leader in pushing the envelope regarding what is possible to achieve through pulmonary rehabilitation and other lifestyle changes in the setting of ILD; an original thinker who is not afraid to challenge conventional wisdom.

In this book, he takes a holistic view of how ILD affects people's lives and psyche. In addition to approaching the subject from the patient's perspective, he takes the unique approach of having patients write many of the chapters in the book. This methodology provides a very fresh and personal vantage point from which to understand and benefit from the first-hand experiences of patients and caregivers, adding further impact to the wealth of practical information contained in this valuable guide to living with ILD.

Respectfully submitted,

Robert J. Kaner, MD
Associate Professor of Clinical and Genetic Medicine
Weill Cornell Medicine
Division of Pulmonary and Critical Care Medicine and
Department of Genetic Medicine

Facilitator's Note by Charlene Marshall, BaSc, MA

The original vision for this book began in late 2019 and feels surreal to finally be holding it in our hands! We, as a group of committed IPF/ILD patients and clinicians, wanted to create a resource that is as unique as your journey with lung disease. As described by Dr. Noah Greenspan, this book is a majestic tapestry; weaving together our personal experiences with IPF/ILD and all the "what-we-wish-we-had-knowns" and "would have-should have-could haves" since our own diagnosis, along with a compilation of information pertinent to the clinical treatment of interstitial lung disease.

As the facilitator for this collective project, I truly believe it is one of the most meaningful projects I will ever work on. The authors of this book literally span the globe and I couldn't be prouder of our efforts to come together, virtually, and regularly to move this project forward. Thinking about what to include in this book took a lot of self-reflection about our own IPF/ILD journey which stirred up emotion. We were vulnerable; sharing our stories with each other and the world but doing so aligned with our vision: making your journey with IPF/ILD easier.

We began this project as a patient group of ten and are finishing it as a group of seven; Don Prager, Tom Hoks and Ann Kelley, we miss you and are grateful for the contributions you made to this book during very difficult times in your lives. With each loss came a shift in personal and group dynamics and the continued decision to keep going after the death of our friends, was like climbing a steep hill, requiring us to keep climbing and pushing ourselves and each other physically and emotionally.

In addition to experiencing loss, our patient group had to contend with many of our own personal issues including social isolation, illness, hospitalizations, transplantation listing, palliative care, and a global Covid pandemic. These adversities caused various bumps in the road throughout the course of our writing process, as did navigating a plethora of different perspectives, personalities, and time zones. Through it all though, the desire to help the IPF/ILD community remained our laser focus and we succeeded in achieving that goal.

To the patient-authors and Dr. Noah Greenspan, who worked tirelessly on this project, you have all inspired me with your colossal efforts, and for that, I will always be grateful to you. Thank you for letting me facilitate this project.

With love,

Charlene Marshall

Editor's Note by Noah Greenspan, PT, DPT, CCS, EMT-B

"The best time to plant a tree is twenty years ago. The second-best time is now." –**Chinese Proverb**

If you are reading this book, it is more than likely that you or someone you know have at one time or another, experienced the sensation of shortness of breath due to respiratory disease. Shortness of breath (SOB), also known as *dyspnea* (pronounced disp-nee-uh) or *air hunger* (pronounced air hun-ger), can be all encompassing and has the potential to undermine every aspect of your life, from the magnificent to the mundane.

There are few sensations in life that are as absolutely terrifying as not being able to catch your breath. In fact, most of us will do absolutely everything in our power to avoid that sensation at all costs, even at the expense of things we love, such as visiting with family and friends; going to the theater, everyday activities such as taking a shower or grocery shopping; even having sex. Shortness of breath can deliver a tremendous blow to our self-esteem as well as our overall quality of life.

Our mission in writing this book is to teach you that for many people, being diagnosed with a chronic respiratory disease is *not* a death sentence and your situation does *not* have to be hopeless, nor should it be. In fact, there are *many* things you can do to *minimize* your shortness of breath as well as to *maximize* your overall health and quality of life.

Our mission in writing this book is *not* to sell you a bill of goods promising a quick fix or cure for your disease or an overnight solution to your shortness of breath. We didn't get here overnight. We're not getting out overnight either. We're also *not* suggesting that managing your disease will be easy. It will not. *But…*if you follow the suggestions in this book, even some of the suggestions, some of the time, you will begin to experience small (and in many cases, not so small) but noticeable improvements in your daily life, whether it be less shortness of breath, the ability to do more of the things you love, increased energy levels, or an improvement in your overall sense of well-being.

Many of the suggestions in this book will work for *many*, if not *most* people reading it. However, it is important to understand that when it comes to patient care and people in general, all of us are different and therefore, need to be treated as individuals. As such, there will always be exceptions to the rule that will require some adjustments or "tinkering" with the methodology.

SOB or *dyspnea on exertion* (DOE) is by far, the single most common presenting symptom of respiratory disease and almost always the symptom that causes people to seek medical attention *and my professional assistance.* However, it is important to note that shortness of breath can also be the consequence of other conditions besides respiratory disease; ranging in severity from the serious, like cardiovascular disease, anemia, or renal disease; to the more benign, but still important-to-address conditions like gastro-esophageal reflux disease (GERD) or deconditioning due to inactivity (i.e., being out of shape); or it could be related to something else entirely.

My point in telling you this is that I don't want you to make any assumptions or self-diagnoses as to the cause of your shortness of breath, without being sure that there aren't other contributing factors that can potentially be harmful to you if left untreated. With that in mind, it is essential that your physician perform a comprehensive workup of your symptoms before beginning any meaningful course of treatment or undertaking any significant lifestyle change *such as cardiopulmonary physical therapy or rehabilitation.*

SOB can range in severity from barely noticeable to all encompassing. At times, you may not even be aware of your symptoms while at others, they may stop you dead (or at least, completely breathless) in your tracks. Depending upon where you are, what you happen to be doing, even who you happen to be with at the time, you may attempt to minimize or make light of your symptoms. You may even tell yourself (and others) little white lies such as: "I'm getting old" or "I'm out of shape" or "It's not a big deal." But you know darn well it is. When I hear people use phrases like "It's not a big deal," I am reminded of that famous river in northeast Africa called: "the Nile." Denial, get it?

Typically, most people first begin to experience shortness of breath at high levels of exertion, during activities such as stair climbing or walking uphill. In New York City, the three things that patients complain about most are climbing subway stairs, walking up the city's many hills and inclines and running *or walking quickly* for the bus; or what we not-so-affectionately like to call "the NYC Pulmonary Triathlon."

Human nature dictates that when we start to experience a certain symptom; any symptom, whether it be shortness of breath, chest pain, back, hip or knee pain; or any other physical (or emotional) distress, we will typically find ways to alleviate or minimize our discomfort; either by modifying the activity that causes us to be symptomatic (e.g. walking more slowly or taking more frequent rest breaks), or by avoiding the activity altogether (e.g. taking a different route or driving, instead of walking uphill or climbing the stairs).

Therein lies *at least part* of the problem. The fact is, once you start to avoid the activities that cause you discomfort (whether they be stair climbing, walking uphill, or running for the bus), all the muscles that you use to perform these activities (including, most importantly, the heart; as well as the respiratory and skeletal muscles), become weaker and more deconditioned. And when muscles become deconditioned, they don't perform as well or use oxygen as efficiently. As a result, you begin to experience shortness of breath at lower levels of activity, and eventually, start to avoid those lower-level activities as well and so on and so on. This is what is known as the *"Dyspnea Cycle."*

In addition to the muscles themselves, all the body systems that are involved in performing these activities also become less efficient and when these systems don't operate as well, guess what. You become *even shorter* of breath at *even lower* levels of activity and in turn, start to avoid *those* activities as well, beginning the cycle all over again. *Sound familiar?*

Patients often describe the *dyspnea cycle* as a "downward spiral," or they tell me that they are "going downhill". The good news is that in the same way that you can "spiral downhill," your body's abilities can actually improve with activity and other positive life-style changes , and in many cases, you can actually start to *"spiral uphill"* again.

At Pulmonary Wellness, whether in person or via our Pulmonary Wellness Bootcamp, the Ultimate Pulmonary Wellness Lecture Series, Ultimate Pulmonary Wellness Facebook Group, or this book, our goal is to help you break this cycle in three ways. First, we will teach you more effective breathing techniques designed to increase your awareness of and give you greater control over your shortness of breath. Second, we will teach you how to exercise, both aerobically (e.g., Walkabouts, treadmill, exercise bike, upper body ergometer, and Arms-Up) and anaerobically (e.g., strength flexibility, and balance training), so that your body becomes stronger and more efficient at using oxygen; and you, less short of breath.

Last, but not least, we will educate you about the various lifestyle factors that play a role in how well or how poorly you breathe, so that you can begin to *reverse* your shortness of breath as well as any other limitations or modifications you've had to make and that have wreaked so much havoc in your life.

With this principle in mind, our purpose in writing this book is *not* to give you a complex list of instructions or fancy protocols that are difficult to understand and virtually impossible to follow. Instead, our goal is to present you with a wealth of information that my patients and I have found to be both successful and practical over the past 30 years.

Again, each person is different, and every situation is unique. Therefore, not all things will work for all people. However, our hope is that this information will help guide you and your health-care team in determining which tools and techniques will work best *for you* and which ones won't be as helpful, or not helpful at all.

As I mentioned earlier, there are few greater teachers than first-hand experience and I am proud to say that the overwhelming majority of what I have learned about pulmonary disease (and its most effective management) has come from my patients (and from watching *House*). I have also been extremely fortunate to be exposed to great instructors and brilliant mentors throughout both my formal education and my professional career but by far, it has been my patients that have been my most instrumental teachers. For that reason (and because Gregory House, MD is a fictional television character), we really wanted this book to be written **with patients, by patients and for patients.**

In sharing our collective experience with you, we hope to give you a direct link to the greatest source of information about your disease, and to help you avoid some of the same pitfalls that others before you have had to deal with. One thing that I can tell you for certain is that even more gratifying than trial and error; is trial and success.

The good news is that most of the information being passed on to you has come directly from the source: ***other patients***. They are the true *experts* in the field, who have experienced many of the same struggles as you *and* found ways to overcome them, even when it seemed like all odds were against them and *you can too*. It is my hope that by putting our collective knowledge and experience together in one comprehensive, yet easy to understand "bible" for pulmonary patients, you will have at your disposal, a wealth of options to choose from, and that you too, will be able to experience your own little slice of "Ultimate Pulmonary Wellness."

Introduction

If you are reading this book, there is a pretty good chance that you or a loved one have been given a diagnosis of Pulmonary Fibrosis (PF), Idiopathic Pulmonary Fibrosis (IPF) or Interstitial Lung Disease (ILD). As if the words themselves aren't complex and scary enough, you are likely left with many feelings and questions about what this means and how a chronic lung disease will affect your health and the rest of your life moving forward. The authors intimately understand this experience completely because at one time or another, we've all been there as we are all pulmonary fibrosis patients ourselves.

As fellow patients *and one rehabilitation specialist in a pear tree*, our mission in writing this book is to share information with you that has collectively taken us decades of research, clinical practice *and firsthand experience* to acquire in the hope of helping you avoid some of the same challenges and pitfalls that we, ourselves have experienced and that we wish someone had been there to tell us when we were first starting out on this rollercoaster that nobody asks to be on.

Note: This book is not a medical book. Rather, it is more of a practical field guide, based on the experiences of a diverse group of people living with PF, IPF or some other form of ILD *and one rehabilitation specialist in a pear tree*. In sharing our experiences with you, we hope to provide you with our best personal advice on how to continue *living* your life, despite a difficult disease. And while not all things will be effective for all people; we ultimately hope to help make your life easier, less stressful, and more enjoyable.

About Us

Before we get down into the weeds or the nitty gritty, we wanted to introduce ourselves and share our own stories with you, so that you can have a better understanding of who we are, where we are coming from, and know that we stand alongside you in solidarity.

Ann

Hello. I am Ann. I am 77 years old, and I have an extensive family network that works together to offer me support in my journey. I live in a small, comfortable neighborhood with neighbors that also keep an eye out for me. I have been a very active person all my life. I was a member of two alumni groups, volunteered for the Salvation Army, and socialized regularly with friends. I also regularly drove 13 hours to visit my grandkids in South Florida.

I had initially begun experiencing increased difficulty with shortness of breath, especially when walking, and one day, I had trouble walking from a luncheon in a large building back to my car. Then it was walking a block with my friends while trying to talk. It was at that point that I knew it was time to go to the doctor.

After visiting my primary care doctor, I was sent to a pulmonologist at a large medical center that had a Center of Excellence
(COE) for pulmonary diseases. Having worked with this group on
research studies, I knew the doctors and staff. It didn't take long to
realize that I was in trouble. After multiple tests, specialty doctor
visits, and a lung biopsy, the ILD team decided I had IPF and that
I needed supplemental oxygen. The delivery of the diagnosis was
not handled well at all. My 21-year-old grandson was with me at
the time and the doctor basically said: "you have IPF, which means
you have 2 to 5 years to live." We were both in complete shock and I
am quite sure that neither of us heard much of anything after that.
This was not a very good way to deliver any diagnosis, especially
one like IPF. When delivering such news, your doctor should set
aside time to explain your diagnosis, available treatment options
and prognosis; and for you to be able to ask questions as you begin
to process this information.

I know so much more and am so much better prepared to handle
this diagnosis *now* than I was then. My family is still very protective but supportive of me continuing to make my own decisions
and live independently. The Covid-19 pandemic has decreased my
activity level dramatically, but with the help of Zoom and various
online support groups, I have reinvented myself and a created a
new, comfortable lifestyle. And yes, I do realize how lucky I am.

Charlene

My IPF journey began in the Spring of 2016 with the sentence: "Charlene, we're sending you to the emergency department." At the time, I had been dealing with a dry cough, breathlessness, and fatigue for nearly nine months. It would be another five months before I was properly diagnosed. Despite these unusual symptoms, I never suspected I'd have a life-threatening lung disease at twenty-eight years old.

I was working in a hospital at the time; an environment that was very conducive to catching infections. I worked long hours and had repeat interactions with patients who were often very sick, and my evenings and weekends were filled with social activities and events; *all given top priority over rest, sleep, and self-care.*

As a result, the physicians I saw about my symptoms seemed unconcerned. After all, I did have age on my side and no underlying health conditions, so it was unlikely that it was anything serious. That changed dramatically in April 2016 when I was diagnosed with IPF.

It took thirteen months to confirm my IPF diagnosis and sadly, based on what I know about other patients' experiences, that isn't unusual. Throughout those thirteen months, the physicians suspected I had everything from adult-onset asthma to chronic bronchitis, to pneumonia, to any one of many various viral or bacterial infections. The symptoms of each of these mirrored how I felt, but the medications typically used to treat those various illnesses were not very effective for me and very soon after finishing a prescribed course of inhalers, steroids, or antibiotics, my breathlessness would return, and the doctors would reconvene.

Like most, I had never heard of IPF, so despite thirteen months of progressively worsening symptoms, I never suspected that I had anything seriously wrong with my lungs. The diagnosing physician (who is no longer responsible for my respiratory care), and I went through numerous potential causes of my PF; household exposures, environmental toxins, recreational activities, second-hand smoke, and genetics, among others, and there was still no glaring reason that could explain my lung damage. Five years later, I still don't have an answer as to why I ended up with IPF and in fact, the word *idiopathic* means exactly that; of unknown cause or origin.

Grace

I think about my IPF diagnosis in two separate stages. The first stage was in 2006; yes, fifteen years ago. I had been unable to shake a chill and had developed a persistent cough that would not clear up despite various medical treatments. I attended a nearby respiratory hospital where I underwent chest X-rays, CT scans and pulmonary function tests. After some deliberation, the consultant there advised me that I was demonstrating signs and symptoms of IPF, which was a chronic, progressive illness; and that no pharmaceutical cure was available.

He suggested that it may be useful to consider long term antibiotics and steroid medication as a preventative measure. I was 65 at the time and had recently retired from my holistic dental practice. I had plans in place to start a new career in permaculture, travel, and spend more time with my new grandchildren, so the "prophylactic approach" did not make much sense to me, not even when the prognostic figures painted that scary picture that I would probably die in 3-5 years.

I just couldn't find the evidence that the suggested that medication would aid in my health or my quality of life. I'd like to say that this was a well-thought-out decision-making process, but in fact, it was my own form of denying both the diagnosis and prognosis, combined with my desire for a healthy a lifestyle. But as you can tell, I am still here.

Approximately five years after my initial diagnosis, I had convinced myself (and possibly even the medical consultant) that the original diagnosis could be wrong. Unfortunately, after rechecking his data, he did confirm that the original diagnosis was correct. Overall, I was ignoring the fact that I was living a life that I *knew* was going to be short but continued doing what I wanted to do and what I had planned to do. Those plans included travelling several times each year to Catalonia and working at an altitude of around 3,500 feet. So far, so good.

The second stage that I refer to didn't begin until several years later. I was working in Catalonia and discovered a reduced ability to walk up the hillside without being short of breath. I was also becoming more tired than normal but despite knowing that I had

IPF, colleagues, family members and I were happy to attribute this to getting older or becoming less fit. But the symptoms remained which eventually convinced me to seek another opinion.

An initial x-ray sought by my primary care doctor was quickly followed up on by the respiratory unit with high resolution CT scan and lung function tests. By this time, I was not feeling well at all. The in-person consultation that followed had the new consultant say that I could not have IPF and that it would be advisable to have an open chest lung biopsy to clarify the diagnosis. I declined that, as I did not believe that I was well enough to cope with such a procedure. A few weeks later as I was starting to feel better, I did agree to a bronchial lavage, at which time, bronchoscopy revealed the presence of Aspergillus (a fungus), and a joint medical team definitively confirmed my diagnosis of IPF.

This second stage was also the beginning of a completely different degree of IPF for me, which was now significantly affecting my lifestyle. At this point, I had become dependent on supplemental oxygen, and it was clear that I was suffering from a progressive illness. Despite being told I had IPF twice, my story highlights the fact that PF can present in different ways for different patients.

John

I developed a severe respiratory infection in early November 2019. However, since I had already been experiencing regular bouts of chronic bronchitis for many (30+) years prior to that, I assumed that I would be able to medicate myself out of this ailment as I had done many times before. At my wife's insistence I went to a walk-in medical clinic in Albany, NY, where the young doctor diagnosed me with pneumonia, prescribed medications, and suggested that I follow up with my general practitioner.

I didn't have a chest X-ray as my visit was on a weekend and naively, I assumed that things would simply get better with the prescribed medications as they had in the past. At a follow-up appointment with my general practitioner, I had a chest X-ray and was contacted two days later informing me that he did not see any evidence of pneumonia, but that he was concerned about the amount of scar tissue in my lungs on the chest X-ray.

My general practitioner referred me to a pulmonologist who I saw in mid-December 2019. They scheduled sleep studies, blood tests, and a CT-scan and I was initially diagnosed with ILD in late January 2020. I had two pulmonary function tests about seven weeks apart and after the second test, I had a virtual appointment with my pulmonologist.

I had several questions about my illness which was now defined as IPF. I asked about my longevity and shared my fears about the information I had found on Dr. Google. My pulmonologist reassured me that I still had a lot more life left in me, and that I shouldn't be so concerned.

However, while my wife and I were speaking with him, his face suddenly changed as he started to review my latest pulmonary function tests. In fact, he seemed almost panicked. He informed me that my lung function had dropped by 26% and he wanted me to start taking a medication called Esbriet as soon as possible. It took an additional seven weeks before I finally started in July 2020. I am currently tolerating the Esbriet medication very well and my team and I believe it has slowed down the progression of my IPF.

Almost immediately after being diagnosed, I joined several IPF support groups and found Noah Greenspan's book, *Ultimate Pulmonary Wellness,* which I read from cover to cover. I did this research and data mining of my own volition. I've made my pulmonologist aware of my involvement with these groups and it was like "oh, good for you," very nonchalant.

Folks, if there is one piece of advice I can share with you, it would be to please keep in mind that *YOU are your own best advocate!*

Linda

Unlike many, my initial diagnosis and care by my pulmonologist was a very positive experience. I had been having trouble breathing for several years and my pulmonary function tests were good, so they kept looking for heart issues. On one particularly hot day, my breathing suddenly became significantly worse, and I took myself to the emergency room. When I arrived, my oxygen saturation was in the low 80's and a CT scan showed scarring in my lungs. I was immediately hospitalized for further evaluation and treatment.

The pulmonologist on call spent time explaining what might be wrong with me. She ordered tests and told me I would need a lung biopsy. Unfortunately, I had complications with the open lung biopsy, but she was able to diagnose me with Hypersensitivity Pneumonitis (another form of ILD) with fibrosis. She treated me for 3 months but when I continued to have exacerbations, she acknowledged that she had very few patients with pulmonary fibrosis and only one with HP.

She suggested I go to a center that specializes in PF and recommended I move out of the area, since my HP appeared to be related to my local environment. She gave me a referral to the Interstitial Lung Disease Center at UCLA. I had family living in the area, so I moved and enrolled as a patient at the center. They changed my medicines and began monitoring my progress. Thankfully, it has been eight years since then and the fibrosis in my lungs has not progressed.

René

I have been in good physical condition all my life. In 2014, I was on an annual ski vacation in Jackson Hole, Wyoming in the USA and found myself considerably out of breath on the slopes. And even worse, my ski buddies were all out-skiing me. I thought to myself, "Well, you *are* getting older, and you *are* high in the mountains where there is less oxygen, that's probably it." But in my heart, I knew that what I was experiencing was not normal.

Back home in Bonaire (Dutch Caribbean), I went to my general practitioner, who sent me to a cardiologist. A stress test was done which revealed a very strong heart. A CT scan was also done, which was deemed "normal." Further testing in 2015 and 2016 yielded the same results; but I still didn't believe it. I was still competing in sporting events but was becoming increasingly short of breath and not performing well at all, even in shorter, less challenging events that I would have easily won in the past.

In 2017 while skiing in Bozeman, Montana; I felt a worsening shortness of breath on the slopes again. My wife took me to a local walk-in medical clinic, and they did chest x-rays and blood tests and within 45 minutes, they told me that I had an ILD. I was told to take Prednisone, continue my vacation, and when I returned home, see a pulmonologist to determine which specific form of interstitial lung disease I had. At this point, I had no idea about the seriousness of my lung disease and naively thought I would get some medicines and it would be gone. However, back home, a CT scan confirmed my ILD.

Due to limited medical facilities in Bonaire, I went to Houston, Texas and had six-weeks of every possible test to see if I had an infectious or autoimmune disease, or one of the other possible alternatives. I was poked, prodded, pinched, jabbed, and turned upside down. I was told that it looked like IPF, but there were also indications of Sarcoidosis, and only a lung biopsy could confirm either one definitively. The lung biopsy was finally done in New York City, and unfortunately my IPF diagnosis was confirmed.

It took months before I realized the seriousness and the consequences of having this relentless, terrifying disease. We then went back over the reports of the previous CT scans and found some definite "snowy white" scarring which was never picked up by my doctors, whose excuse was that "IPF is very difficult to diagnose." I lost four years that I should have been on the anti-fibrosis medications. Sadly, this is not uncommon when dealing with a disease like IPF, which is one of our major motivators in writing this book.

Ronald

In the spring of 2017, at my annual physical exam, my family doctor spent an unusual amount of time listening to my lungs. He reported hearing a "crackling" sound. A chest X-ray followed shortly, and then a CT scan of my lungs. Shortly thereafter, my family doctor called to say that he thought I most likely had IPF, and that he wanted to refer me to a pulmonologist he knew and respected. At the time, I was 68, and had never heard of IPF before.

Even though we live in a rural area of Canada, a pulmonologist visits our local office four days a month. I must say that our first appointment was a little rough. As he scrolled down through my CT scan, he kept muttering: "oh, that's bad," which was far from reassuring. He thought that it was likely IPF but said I would need more tests to be sure.

During our second appointment, we discussed supplemental oxygen. When I asked him what criteria he used to determine when oxygen was needed, he answered with a patronizing comment to the effect of "doctor knows best." That response really raised my hackles (which is very unusual for me). But I have a science background and want to understand the factors behind certain decisions, and I fully expected to have input before any decisions about *my* treatment were made.

But that little tiff changed everything about our relationship. I came to understand that many of his patients were quite happy to just have the doctor tell them what to do. And he understood that while I appreciated his knowledge and advice, I wanted to maintain control of decisions affecting my health. Thankfully, our relationship warmed considerably after that and now, our discussions are much more collegial, I receive copies of all my test results, and we both feel much more comfortable with each other.

One of the items we discussed was the difficulty in making a definitive diagnosis of IPF since the "honeycomb patterns" in my lungs were indistinct. We talked about the possibility of a lung biopsy but neither of us wanted that. Instead, he recommended I get a second opinion from the Toronto Lung Clinic. Each of our visits to Toronto began with a pulmonary function test and a six-minute walk test to measure how my blood oxygen level responded to exertion. They sent me to a rheumatologist as well to rule out lupus, and I had an echocardiogram to make sure there was no heart damage present.

Toronto's conclusions were basically the same as our home pulmonologist; that this is likely IPF, which seems to be about as firm a diagnosis as you can expect. Luckily, my family doctor identified my diagnosis correctly within the first few weeks. The next six months were spent ruling out other possibilities and more definitively confirming IPF as the culprit. IPF is now a central part of my life.

Ruth

When I first started to suspect something was wrong, I had been having severe shortness of breath walking from the parking garage to my office, which was only a block away. I knew I was out of shape, but thought to myself, "this is ridiculous." My first thought was to go to a cardiologist, since my parents had both had heart issues. After the cardiologist gave me a clean bill of heart health, I saw a pulmonologist next. During childhood, I had often experienced long and severe bouts of bronchitis but never thought much of it. Among a whole bunch of other tests, he ordered a High-Resolution CT (HRCT) scan.

I was on vacation with friends when I got a voicemail from my doctor that said: "Mrs. O'Bryan, we have gotten the results of your HRCT scan and we need to talk. It's not an emergency but I'll call you later." I waited a day and a half, and finally called his office and said: "I need to talk to the doctor immediately, he's ruining my vacation!" A short time later, I got a call back from the doctor who said: "If it looks like a duck, walks like a duck and quacks like a duck, it's a duck. You have Pulmonary Fibrosis."

My doctor had suspected IPF in 2012 but waited until March 2016 to order a lung biopsy to determine exactly what kind of fibrosis I had. The results in the report stated that I had Usual Interstitial Pneumonia (UIP). I had no idea what I was dealing with at the time.

Fortunately, I made the decision to go to a pulmonary doctor who practices at an ILD Center of Excellence (COE). Sadly, many people are not diagnosed (or are often misdiagnosed) until they are in the later stages of their disease. This is one of the reasons that we see it as our mission to help raise awareness and educate others about pulmonary fibrosis and other interstitial lung diseases so patients and doctors can act quickly with respect to both diagnosis and treatment.

What We've Learned

As you can see, each of us arrived at our respective diagnoses in different ways. The timeline varied drastically for each of us, along with the way in which we were told about our disease and the tests used to rule out other ailments before arriving at a definitive diagnosis. Suffice to say, we all wish the diagnostic journey was clearer and more consistent and hope that by sharing our experiences, we can help make the journey a little easier for our fellow patients. Please know that you are not alone. We are here for you and hope that this book will provide you with some valuable insights and information that will make your experiences smoother than ours.

Chapter 1:

Shortness of Breath by Noah Greenspan, PT, DPT, CCS, EMT-B

Typically, when people first begin to experience shortness of breath or dyspnea on exertion (DOE), they either find ways to modify the activities that cause them discomfort, or they simply avoid them altogether. While this may seem like the safest and most reasonable course of action, lowering your activity level can worsen the situation, causing you to become weaker and shorter of breath over time, until even life's simplest tasks, like showering or getting dressed, can become difficult thanks to *that miserable SOB (shortness of breath).*

Let's use stair climbing as an example. In our small town of New York City, our subway steps are not built for comfort. Rather, they are designed for efficiency, which here in New York City means "space-saving." As a result, they are usually longer, higher, and steeper than the stairs in most people's homes or even those you might encounter in a restaurant or movie theater. Add to this scenario, a mob of type-A New Yorkers during rush hour, and the situation more closely resembles the running of the bulls than a daily commute. Patients frequently tell me that they don't take the subway anymore because they can no longer climb the stairs. Instead, they take the bus or taxi, or Access-A-Ride, (but that's a whole 'nother story, altogether).

Again, using our stair-climbing example, think about how much less activity a person will get if they switch from taking the subway to taking the bus. Let's say they usually commute to work five days per week and have two flights of stairs going to work and two flights coming back home. That's 20 flights of stairs per week—80 flights per month—and nearly 1000 flights per year.

It isn't hard to imagine that if you climb 1000 fewer flights of stairs this year than you did last year, your body will naturally (or more accurately, *unnaturally*), become less conditioned, and you will likely experience an increase in your shortness of breath. Incidentally, these negative adaptations to inactivity can happen even if you don't have a pulmonary disease.

Now, here is a concept that is very important to understand. The inability to climb stairs can be affected by many factors including shortness of breath, cardiovascular disease, muscle weakness or fatigue. It can even be caused by anxiety, which, incidentally, is both increased by shortness of breath and increases shortness of breath (*another vicious cycle we want to break*). Or it can be cause by osteoarthritis or spinal stenosis or *something else altogether.*

But, as you become more deconditioned, one consequence is that your body does not use oxygen as efficiently. As a result, you then start to feel short of breath at lower levels of activity. Then, you start to avoid *those* (even lower level) activities, and so on and so forth. Again, this is called *the dyspnea cycle* or *dyspnea spiral* and our goal is to help you break that cycle by teaching you more effective breathing techniques—and teaching you how to exercise *most* effectively every time, so that your body becomes more efficient at using oxygen and you, more fit and less short of breath.

For many people, their symptoms can get so bad that the activity doesn't seem possible or worth the effort anymore. Depending upon where you live and the resources available to you, this scenario can drastically limit the things you can do, the places you can go, and the people you can see. We will also discuss some of the challenges of portable oxygen use later in the book.

Some of my patients can map out the city by where there are steep (or in some cases, not so steep) inclines or hills. Others can map out the city based on where there are places to sit down and rest, and still others, by the availability of public restrooms. They take the easier routes whenever possible and avoid hills like the plague. But as you might have guessed, all the muscles that they use to walk uphill become deconditioned, and they now start to feel short of breath at even lower levels of activity (e.g., walking on flat surfaces). *Sound familiar?*

There is also another important possibility that you (and your doctor) should consider. Believe it or not, it is completely possible that your shortness of breath could be the result of something else altogether. Patients come to me all the time that can't understand why they're shorter of breath. "Nothing has changed," they protest. That's when I start my interrogation. I inquire knowingly as to whether there have been any changes in their medications, exercise regimen, weight, and etcetera, etcetera.

"Oh, yeah. I have gained (or lost) a little weight," they say. To which I say: "How much? "About 25 pounds," they say (or 30, or 40, or more). To which I say: "So, you've gained 25 (or lost 10) pounds and think nothing's changed?"

Let me put this in perspective for you: 25 pounds is the equivalent of two bowling balls. Try carrying two bowling balls around with you all day, every day, for a while. I am pretty sure that you will get tired more easily, have more difficulty climbing stairs, and yes; feel shorter of breath. And when you lose 10 pounds without trying, there is a good chance that at least some, if not most of that is muscle.

We'll discuss the subject of weight in greater detail in the nutrition chapter, but my point in introducing it now, is to illustrate that there are many factors besides the lungs and the respiratory system that contribute to breathing and consequently, SOB.

At Pulmonary Wellness, our goal is to help patients break this "dyspnea cycle" by teaching them more effective breathing techniques and exercising them most effectively, so that their bodies become more efficient at using oxygen. We also *educate* our patients about their disease, medications, the benefits of exercise, eating healthy, managing stress and anxiety, and the pitfalls of cigarette smoking and inactivity. I truly believe that in most cases, an educated patient will be a healthier (and happier) patient.

A well-known principle in medical ethics is *"Primum Non Nocere."* This phrase comes from the Latin, meaning, *"First, do no harm."* At our Center, patient safety is our first, second, and third priority.

We believe in a "no-setback" approach to cardiopulmonary rehabilitation and when it comes to patient care, I don't like surprises. That's why everything we do at the Center is done under fully monitored conditions.

As our rehabilitation patients exercise, they are "telemetrically monitored", which is a fancy way of saying that they wear an electrocardiogram (ECG), so that we can continuously monitor their heart rate and rhythm during exercise. Their blood pressure and oxygen saturation are each measured in 5-minute increments. Again, our patients' safety is our first, second, and third priority.

The beauty of this type of monitoring system is that we can be confident in adjusting our patients' programs, not just daily, but even within each individual workout, allowing us to ensure not only their safety, but also that they are receiving the maximum benefit from every session. This methodology is the real secret to our success, *and of course, the karaoke.*

Most recently, we have developed an at-home cardiopulmonary "bootcamp," to allow you to stay in touch, get educated and get in your exercise even if you don't have access to a formal, in-person rehabilitation program. Bootcamp aims to take all our experience of the past 30 years and bring it to you form the comfort of your home, or anywhere else in the world. We will discuss Bootcamp more in the exercise chapter.

Please feel free to share this information with your healthcare team and please be sure to get your doctor's go-ahead before beginning *any* exercise program or implementing *any* lifestyle change. And who knows? He or she may even learn a thing or two that can help his, her, or their other patients.

Finally, your attitude is essential. I understand that when you feel sick, it can be difficult to focus on being shiny, happy, and positive. However, constantly focusing on your illness or all the things you *can't* do can have a profoundly negative impact on your health and well-being. Throughout this book, we will be guiding you and sharing methods that will help you work your way back to wellness, so that your actions and thoughts can begin to have a profoundly *positive* impact on your health and well-being—in other words, *your life*. Don't worry about the starting line. For now, think of yourself as the healthiest you can be *today*…and then get ready to become healthier.

Chapter 2:

Interstitial Lung Diseases by Noah Greenspan, PT, DPT, CCS, EMT-B

This chapter is based upon Ultimate Pulmonary Wellness Webinar 18: "Interstitial Lung Diseases" and "Pulmonary Fibrosis and ILD's: Early Diagnosis and Best Treatments" both with my friend, Robert Kaner, MD; the person who I consider to be one of, if not the tippy-top super guru in Pulmonary Fibrosis (PF), Idiopathic Pulmonary Fibrosis (IPF), and other Interstitial Lung Diseases (ILD's).

The subject of Interstitial Lung Diseases (ILD's) is an extremely complex topic, often even for clinicians, even for physicians, and *even* for many pulmonary specialists. So, it is no surprise that it is equally if not more difficult for patients and other laypeople.

When it comes to ILD's, there is a lot of misunderstanding, misinformation, and confusion out there; so much so, that before we even get into the material, I want to highlight three key points right here from the get-go, because failing to appreciate these concepts can literally mean the difference between life and death.

If you take nothing else away from or don't understand *anything* else in this chapter, please understand the following three points:

1. *Early diagnosis* and *treatment* are critical; especially since some of the ILD's are noted to have a 3-5-year life expectancy

from time of onset, although please don't get hung up on those specific numbers since one, there is variability in these numbers and two, new treatments are being worked on all the time.

2. Getting a *definitive diagnosis* is critical to your care. *One of* the reasons for this is that some of the treatments used to treat *some* ILD's have not only been proven ineffective; but they can be harmful in the case of other ILD's, meaning that they can make the disease worse by speeding up its progression.

3. Having the right team, especially, a pulmonologist who *specializes* in ILD's is also critical. ILD's are serious and cannot afford to be handled by anything less than an expert. I would say "as serious as cancer", but in many cases, ILD can be more serious in some cases, so only the best and the brightest will do.

If you do not have access to physicians and other health care professionals that specialize in ILD's then you need to find one, even if it means travelling to an academic medical center or Center of Excellence in another location. In doing so, you can be properly diagnosed and started on the right treatment regimen. Then, after getting a definitive diagnosis and initial treatment plan, you can be managed along with your local pulmonologist. Again, this can literally be the difference between life and death.

Please understand that I am not telling you these things to scare the bejesus out of you. Chances are, that's already been done. I am telling you these things to impress upon you the fact that ILD is nothing to play with, nothing to sleep on, and not something to dabble with. You cannot afford *not* to take this seriously. And if

you choose to stop reading here, *"get thee to an ILD specialist, go."*
-William Shakespeare (partially)

When people talk about obstructive lung diseases like Asthma, Emphysema, or Chronic Bronchitis, which are diseases that affect the *airways*, most people have at least a *general* idea of what we're talking about. But...when you say the words "interstitial lung disease" or "ILD," people generally have *no idea* what you're talking about (again, including many clinicians). So, in the interest of getting us off on the right foot, let's talk about what ILD's are, what they aren't; and why they are so difficult to diagnose and treat.

To be clear, ILD is not one specific disease or diagnosis. Rather, ILD's are a large *group* of disorders; or more specifically, a category or classification of diseases, that are grouped together because they have similar clinical, radiographic (X-ray or CT scan), and pathological mechanisms.

Anatomy and Physiology

Interstitial lung diseases occur in the alveoli, or alveolar spaces, where gas exchange occurs. Deep within this gas-exchanging part of the lungs, there is an interface between the capillaries, where red blood cells take on oxygen from outside to be used by the body and release carbon dioxide to the atmosphere. The alveolus is surrounded by a very thin structure, called the alveolar wall, which contains epithelial cells that line the air space; and pulmonary capillaries that are only wide enough to accommodate one red blood cell at a time. There is also a connective tissue "scaffolding" that holds that structure together. Interstitial lung diseases are centered on those alveolar walls and the structures that hold the gas exchanging part of the lung together.

Often, people will compare the alveoli to a bunch of grapes. So, if you think of a cluster of alveoli as a bunch of grapes, the alveolar wall would be analogous to the skin of the grape, and that's what gives it its tensile strength and the ability to maintain its structure. So, the simple explanation is that when you have an interstitial lung disease, the skin of the grape gets thicker, and you end up with smaller grapes with less air in each grape.

But it turns out that the physiology is a little bit more complicated. In a normal lung, you have this very thin membrane that allows oxygen to go from the airspace of the lung into the pulmonary capillary. In a normal lung, the distance that the oxygen must travel to cross that membrane is very short. In the case of ILD, this membrane gets thicker and the distance for diffusion is longer, so the process is going to be less efficient, but it turns out to be even more complex than that. I told you it's complex!

Think of your pulmonary circulation as a series of parallel pipes. Your entire cardiac output, i.e., the volume of blood pumped by your heart, must travel through these pipes, aka the pulmonary circulation and when we exercise, this cardiac output increases dramatically. In a person with normal, healthy lungs, there is enough capacity in these pipes to allow for this increased cardiac output to travel through the pulmonary circulation effectively.

However, when you have a progressive interstitial lung disease, there's inflammation and scarring in the gas exchanging part of the lung, and over time, you lose more and more of those pipes. In this situation, the only way you can maintain cardiac output is for the velocity of the red cells to increase, so they start speeding through the remaining pulmonary capillaries faster and faster.

Again, in a person with normal, healthy lungs, the red blood cell is in the pulmonary capillary for about a quarter of a second, and by the time it goes from the beginning of the capillary to the end, it's completely saturated with oxygen. However, if you lose enough of your pulmonary circulation, the red blood cells may have to go so fast during either exercise or activity, that they are unable to become fully saturated with oxygen by the time they get to the end. This is known as exercise-induced oxygen desaturation, and the more capillaries you lose, the worse it gets, as interstitial lung disease progresses.

Therefore, in people that have interstitial lung disease, their oxygen saturation at rest may be perfectly normal or near normal, but when they exercise, their oxygen saturation drops, sometimes very dramatically and that's why you may need large amounts of supplemental oxygen when you exercise to compensate for that impaired physiology.

Getting the Right Diagnosis

One experience that we hear from people repeatedly is that they've seen "X number of doctors," or they've been short of breath "for X number of years," and somehow, they still don't get diagnosed with IPF or interstitial lung disease. It's actually very common that there's a lag, sometimes a long lag, between the time people first develop symptoms to getting to a diagnosis of interstitial lung disease, and there are several reasons for that. As you read in the introductions, when people initially develop exertional symptoms, they often chalk them up to being older or deconditioned or maybe having a heart problem or something else altogether, and often, their primary care physician may view it in much the same way, so they may go through an extensive cardiac workup before anyone even considers checking the lungs.

Another reason is that up until very recently, at least for Idiopathic Pulmonary Fibrosis, there weren't any pharmacological treatments available for IPF, so some physicians seem to have taken the position of "well, there's nothing I can do about the disease anyway, so what's the point of looking for it?" Well, now there are several things we can do, so there *definitely is a point* in looking for it, and since we know that early diagnosis and treatment is crucial, we would encourage anyone who has unexplained respiratory symptoms to have them investigated.

Diagnosing ILD would be much simpler if we knew for sure, what symptoms we're looking for. We would be able to tell patients, caregivers, and clinicians, "if you see this, this and this, think interstitial lung disease."

However, part of the complexity in recognizing ILD, is that most of the symptoms are non-specific for interstitial lung disease. In other words, the main symptoms people experience early in interstitial lung disease, such as cough and shortness of breath on exertion can occur with other diseases like asthma or COPD, Congestive Heart Failure, or Pulmonary Hypertension, among others. In fact, there are a whole host of diseases that can cause those exact same symptoms.

So, it's helpful to have an attentive physician who can try to sort out which category of disease is causing those problems, and that may involve various kinds of testing. These include a careful history, a good physical exam and some basic tests like a chest x-ray and an echocardiogram. When there's a suspicion of interstitial lung disease, it's very important to get a CT scan of the chest, and it needs to be done in a very specific way. For suspected ILD, it's important to have a high-resolution CT scan (HRCT).

A conventional CT scan gives you images of individual slices of lung tissue that are about 5 millimeters in thickness. To properly diagnose interstitial lung disease, a high-resolution CT scan is required, in which the individual slices are about 1.25 millimeters in thickness or thinner.

Another difference is that during a conventional chest CT, all the images are taken during inspiration. However, when ILD is suspected, images are also taken during expiration. Comparing the two helps to identify a phenomenon called air trapping, which occurs in interstitial lung diseases where there is obstruction of the small airways. This typically occurs in conditions like chronic hypersensitivity pneumonitis, which is a very important category of ILD's, and you may not be able to make that diagnosis any other way.

Classification

We know that there are a lot of patients who are living in places where they don't have access to an academic teaching hospital or COE, and they may not even have access to a pulmonary doctor. In fact, we hear from people all the time that say, "I've been going to my doctor, and I've been telling him (or her or they) I have a cough and I'm short of breath and still no diagnosis."

Again, interstitial lung disease is confusing to a lot of physicians and it's even confusing to pulmonary specialists because ILD patients make up a small minority of the total number of patients that the average pulmonologist would see, and it's a very confusing area of medicine, both for diagnosis and treatment. And again, since the most expertise in both diagnosis and treatment of interstitial lung disease is typically concentrated in academic medical centers, for people who have those symptoms, and don't have a definitive diagnosis yet, it might be worth their while to make the trip to at least get the right diagnosis, and then they can be put on the right path to follow up back at home with their own doctors.

ILD's can be divided into two broad categories:

1. ILD's with Known Causes
2. ILD's with Unknown Causes (Idiopathic)

ILD's with Known Causes include:

- Occupational Lung Disease
- Hypersensitivity Pneumonitis
- Autoimmune and Connective Tissue Disorders
- Pneumonia and Other Infections
- Drugs/Medications that cause Pulmonary Toxicity
- Other Known Causes

Occupational Lung Diseases

Occupational lung diseases are caused by exposures to toxic, inorganic dust that people breathe in, usually while they're working, such as asbestos, silica, coal, among others. These include conditions like *Asbestosis* and *Coal Worker's Pneumoconiosis* (Black Lung Disease). If someone is diagnosed with Occupational Lung Disease, the first order of business is that they discontinue that exposure as difficult as that may be for many.

Hypersensitivity Pneumonitis

Hypersensitivity Pneumonitis is caused by breathing in *organic* dust or antigens such as mold, fungal spores, or bird antigens, for people who keep birds as pets. A lot of times people with HP may not even be aware that there's mold in their home. As an example, maybe they had a flood years ago and the water was cleaned up, but they didn't realize that there was mold growing behind the drywall or in their basement.

For people that are in a very early stage of HP where the predominant pathology in their lungs is inflammation, they can expect to see a big improvement in their lung disease once the trigger is removed. On the other hand, if they already have advanced lung disease where there's already a lot of scar tissue (fibrosis) involved, their symptoms and lung function might stabilize, but it might not improve substantially. Again, yet another case for early diagnosis and treatment.

Autoimmune and Connective Tissue Disorders as a cause of ILD

Another big category of diseases is those that are associated with systemic connective tissue disorders. Examples of common CTD's include Rheumatoid Arthritis, Lupus, Scleroderma, Sjogren's Syndrome, Dermatomyositis, Polymyositis, Anti-Synthetase Syndrome, Rheumatoid Arthritis, and others.

Pneumonia as a cause of ILD

In some cases, ILD can be caused by severe cases of bacterial, viral, or fungal infections.

Medications as a cause of ILD

Some medications can cause pulmonary toxicity leading to ILD. The most common ones include *bleomycin*, which is used for chemotherapy and *amiodarone*, which is used for a variety of cardiac conditions including Atrial Fibrillation.

ILD's with Unknown Causes include:

- Non-Specific Interstitial Pneumonia (NSIP)
- Idiopathic Pulmonary Fibrosis (IPF)
- Other Unknown Causes

Non-Specific Interstitial Pneumonia (NSIP)

The other broad category is idiopathic interstitial lung diseases, in which the cause is completely unknown. In this case, they must be correctly classified. One classification is called **non-specific interstitial pneumonia** (NSIP), which is a completely misleading term. For one, there *are* specific criteria for diagnosing it, and it's *not* an infection. It's an inflammatory disease.

Idiopathic Pulmonary Fibrosis

The other classification is ***Idiopathic Pulmonary Fibrosis (IPF)***, the most common interstitial lung disease of unknown cause. IPF is diagnosis of both inclusion and exclusion, meaning first, all other cause must be ruled out and then the inclusive part is to have definitive evidence of usual interstitial pneumonia (UIP) pattern in the lung.

In both NSIP and IPF, a surgical lung biopsy is often the only way to make a definitive diagnosis and since there are major differences between NSIP and IPF with respect to their clinical characteristics, prognosis, and treatment, it's extremely important.

Chapter 3:

Words of Wisdom for the Caregiver by Ruth O'Bryan

Caring for a loved one with a chronic illness can be one of the most stressful and challenging roles of your life – and believe it or not, one of the most gratifying. No one is born intrinsically knowing how to take care of someone with a medical condition, especially one as serious and complex as pulmonary fibrosis. Nor is there any way to be fully prepared if you find yourself in this position.

Even if you do have some degree of medical training, caring for a loved one is not the same as caring for someone under your professional charge. In a professional medical setting, you typically have a support team to back you up when needed, and at the end of your shift, you get to go home. This is not the case when the person who is sick is your significant other, or parent, child, or anyone else whose well-being you have an intimate and vested interest in.

My name is Ruth, and I was a caregiver to my husband for 15 years while he fought prostate cancer. After he died, I was told that he lived at least seven years longer than he would have if not for the "pit bull with lipstick" (me), making sure he got the best care available. During that time, I was also balancing a full-time job with preparing our meals, keeping up with the household tasks, and helping my husband with his basic medical care and other personal needs. Three years later, I was diagnosed with idiopathic pulmonary fibrosis (IPF) – which means that I write this chapter as someone who has walked both sides of the street.

Early in Your Journey

A diagnosis of pulmonary fibrosis, and all that that encompasses, is likely to lead to many challenges and changes in your life; and believe it or not, maybe even some unexpected opportunities. These may include personal, professional, physical, emotional, social, spiritual, financial, practical, and logistical; like writing this book, for example.

Throughout your journey, the most important thing by far that you can do for your loved one is to let them know that you love them and that you are there to support them in whatever way you can. This can include helping them with practical or logistical tasks like going to the doctor with them, listening, asking questions, and taking notes, helping them with their medications, and "intangibles," like simply being there to listen.

Note: For the duration of this chapter, I will use the collective "you" to refer to both you and your partner since so many of things we will discuss are personal and can vary from person to person, couple to couple, family to family, and team to team. In addition, what affects the patient affects all involved and vice versa.

Initially, one of the most important tasks you will need to do is to assemble your care team. Although every care team is unique, yours will likely be comprised of you, your significant other (where applicable) and your loved ones, as well as a bevy of doctors: primary care, cardiology, gastroenterology, and of course, your pulmonary doctor. There may also be other specialists and or ancillary team members, depending upon your own unique personal situation.

Communicate, Communicate, Communicate

Honest, caring, and open communication between patient and caregiver is critical. Forming a partnership and taking the time to evaluate each members roles will be an important early step in your relationship. Assist your loved one in identifying how he, she, or they want to contribute to the care plan, encouraging them to maintain as much control, freedom, and autonomy as possible. Each of you should identify and communicate your strengths and be honest about where you may need assistance.

Feeling that you are continuing to contribute to each other's lives in a meaningful way is important for both of your mental and emotional health, as well as the patient/caregiver relationship. Let each other know how important they are and that they are still a valuable member of your family and community.

One important step you can take that will benefit both you and your loved one is to learn as much as you can about the disease including symptoms, and common medical tests and treatments including potential benefits and side effects. Keep in mind that just because it's on the internet, doesn't make it true or current or even safe, so please be sure to use trusted sources like your doctor and your health care team.

Staying Organized

Whether you are the patient or you're the one caring for someone else, you are often required to keep track of *a lot* of information. There are many ways that this can be done, depending on your personal preferences and how tech-savvy you may or not be.

Personally, I have found that even in this so-called "paperless society," paper can still come in handy. One thing that I found helpful was getting a large 3-ring binder complete with front and back pockets, and a three-hole punch to keep your information tidy.

Include a list of important phone numbers (even if you already have them programmed into your phone). Include the names and contact information of all the doctors and other health care professionals on your team, as well as friends and relatives. I have also found it helpful to keep a chronological list of medical visits and the "goings-on" of those visits including any test results or medication changes.

And speaking of which, keep a *current* list of medications. I've had to call EMS several times for both my husband and I, and your list of medications is always one of the first things they ask for. It can be difficult to remember things during an emergency, and emergency professionals are trained to look for a copy of your medications and medical history on your refrigerator door for easy access.

These days, most hospitals and health-care facilities offer an electronic health record or online "MyChart," which links all hospitals and doctors, so any new medical personnel can view the patient's history (while also saving a few trees in the process). If you prefer, you can also print out hard copies of the most important items to put in your notebook. Wink wink!

Your Feelings Matter Too

As a caregiver, it is very natural to experience a wide range of emotions. Some of the more common feelings caregivers may experience are sadness, anxiety, depression, guilt, or for lack of a better term, the desire to "fix" their loved one and make things all better. It is not uncommon for some caregivers to want to control the course of action or treatment plan. Overcontrolling can be a natural reaction to fear or stress. However, as difficult as it may be, try your best to be supportive and respectful of your loved one's wishes without trying to force them to do what *you* think is right.

The Child Caregiver for a Parent: A Reverse Role

I was a caregiver to my mother before I was a caregiver to my husband. Helping a parent who may still see you as the child can be very difficult for both of you. For one, no matter how old you get, you will always be *their* child, but it is okay to say, "*Please allow me to help take care of you the best I can.*"

Caring for a parent can be similar, yet different to that of a spouse or significant other. There may be days when you aren't sure if you are the child, or the parent/caregiver. It's important to try to be as flexible and open-minded as possible.

On the good days, your parent may feel good and want to do things for themselves. Let them. At other times, they may be worn out or frustrated. That's when you can shift into caregiver mode and be there to help. As discussed earlier, communication is key. Ask them what you can do for them to help make them feel better, establishing and respecting boundaries *together*.

Be on the Lookout for Burnout

As unfair as it may seem, don't be surprised if people rarely ask how *you*, the caregiver are doing. Often, when there is a sick family member, much of the attention can be focused on that person and sometimes, people can forget or not even realize how tough the situation can be on the caregiver. Remind them (and yourself) that you are also a person with your own feelings, stressors, and fears, and nobody can be expected to be strong all the time. In the interest of self-care (or self-preservation), it is perfectly fine and even encouraged to let others know when you need some support.

The Cleveland Clinic defines "Caregiver Burnout" as "a state of physical, emotional and mental exhaustion [that] may be accompanied by a change in attitude, from positive and caring to negative and unconcerned." "Burnout can occur when caregivers do not get the help they need, or if they push themselves to do more than they are truly capable of."

The symptoms of caregiver burnout can be like stress and depression including feeling sad, blue, irritable, hopeless, and helpless; withdrawal from family and friends; loss of interest in social activities or hobbies; changes in appetite, weight loss or gain; and changes in sleep patterns among others. If you are exhibiting any of these signs, please seek the support you need, from family, friends, support groups, your doctor, and in some scenarios, a mental health professional. *Remember that you count too!*

I will admit that while my husband was sick, I didn't take the best care of myself. For years, my doctors would ask me, *"What do you do for you?"* My answer was always *"Nothing, I don't have time for me."* Now I realize how flawed my perception was. The fact is constant stress will eventually take its toll on your body. I sometimes wonder if having been diagnosed with IPF didn't have something to do with the stress I was under for 15 years that I never addressed. Again, finding ways to alleviate your own stress is crucial to the well-being of any caregiver and ultimately, benefits the patient, too.

For managing your own stress, you can utilize one or more of the various mindfulness and meditation techniques readily available in a variety of formats including live, virtual, apps and many others.

Here is one example:

Close your eyes and imagine yourself in a serene, happy place where you are comfortable and at peace. Let your mind go, if only for a few minutes. I like to close my eyes and envision myself at the beach, where I sit in a chair with my feet in the water, letting the waves cascade over them as they break on the shoreline. Try to focus on the things that are truly important to you and cast all other thoughts and worries away.

Donnie Vapor, a colorful musician and one of our co-authors, was an inspiration to all those who knew him. He was always finding new and creative ways to maintain a positive attitude and to truly *live his life* with this disease. He shared this wonderful relaxation technique with us, and I am sharing it with you here in his honor:

If you find your mind racing, visualize a dandelion with all those white, fuzzy seeds. Think about dispersing all your worries onto those soft, billowing seeds. Then, imagine yourself blowing on the seeds and blowing away all your worries with them. Stay there for as long as you want, blowing those seeds, blowing, blowing, as you watch your negative thoughts and worries drifting off into the air.

Another technique that many find helpful is Praying to a Higher Power. One of the most beloved prayers is the Serenity Prayer of St. Francis, which is a prayer for peace: *"God grant me the serenity to accept the things I cannot change, the courage to change the things I can, and the wisdom to know the difference."* Regardless of your religious affiliation or lack thereof, this advice seems to make good sense.

Stay Healthy!

Eat a nutritious diet, drink plenty of water, and try to get in *at least* a little exercise each day. This doesn't mean you have to run a marathon. Walk in your neighborhood, ride a bicycle, do some yoga or Pilates, or if you have access to a pool, try swimming or taking a water aerobics class. If you need a little break, ask a friend or family member to step in so you can have some much needed "me (you) time." Remember, if you're not feeling

well, you won't be much help to anyone else.

Keep A Journal

Journaling can be a very helpful therapeutic release for both patients and caregivers because you're able to express your deepest thoughts and feelings without worrying about what others may think or feel. This is for you and you alone unless you choose to share it with someone else. Many people are pleasantly surprised at how much better they feel after a journaling session.

Join A Group

Consider attending a support group meeting for caregivers. These groups can be very powerful and empowering, providing education and support for and from others who are going through the same or similar experiences. Sometimes, they are the only ones who can truly understand how you feel because they too are "walking the walk." This validation can be invaluable for your emotional, cognitive, and physical well-being.

Seek Professional Help When Needed

There are times when your situational stressors and emotions can feel like they are too much to bear. In this case, it is important to seek the assistance of a mental health professional. There is no shame in asking for help. In fact, it's a sign of strength.

Everyday Challenges

One of the biggest challenges for the caregiver and patient is dealing with your frustrations at not being able to do the things you used to do, as well as the stress and anxiety that accompanies shortness of breath. Try to work through these feelings together by focusing on the here and now and again, again, again, please don't hesitate to seek the help of a mental health professional if things become too tough to bear on your own.

Accentuate the Positive!

Even when faced with a chronic illness, there are still many ways you can maximize the quality of your lives, and with a little creativity, you may even be able to have a little fun in the process. Here are some ideas for fun, meaningful activities you can try:

- **Make a Bucket List!** Include some of the things that you've always wanted to do but still haven't gotten around to...*and do some of them!*
- **Share Your Stories with Family and Friends!** I have written something for my children and grandchildren called...*"The Book of Ruth."*
- **Go Through Those Old Photographs!** Scan them into your computer and hit the "share" button. Label them so when your family members go through them, they won't be saying, *"who the heck is that?"*
- **Movie Night!** Watch a favorite movie with family or friends. Add a little comedy. They say laughter is the best medicine... *and don't forget the popcorn!*
- **Don't Give Up the Things You Love!** Enjoy as much as many and as often possible. Ann, one of the contributors told me that even folding laundry made her feel like she was still able to contribute to her own life. How about knitting or needlepoint, playing cards, or whatever it is that makes you uniquely who you are? *You, Do You!*
- Be a Tourist in Your Own City. Visit the places you have planned to go but never took the time to do so.

Insert YOUR ideas here:

1.

2.

3.

4.

5.

You Are Not Alone

Our hope is that this chapter was helpful to you and your loved ones. In it, I tried to give you some insight, suggestions, tools, and advice that we all wished we had known about while we were struggling to find answers. And if you think of any good ideas, please feel free to share them with us!

We wish you and yours the very best!

Chapter 4:

The Respiratory System by Noah Greenspan, PT, DPT, CCS, EMT-B

KNOW THYSELF!

When it comes to dealing with a chronic illness, a *basic* understanding of the anatomy (structure), physiology (function) and pathophysiology (disease) will go a long way. My hope is that this information will help you better understand your condition, as well as provide you with the necessary vocabulary and context for more meaningful communication with your doctors and other health care professionals.

Breathing is "Multi-Factorial"

I tell people repeatedly that *"breathing is a multi-factorial process."* What I mean by that is that on any given day, there are a whole host of factors, both internal and external to our bodies that can affect how well (or how poorly) we breathe. Besides just our lungs and the respiratory system, these can include things like proper medication use, activity versus inactivity, the foods we eat (or don't eat), maintaining a healthy weight as compared to being overweight or underweight and managing stress and anxiety effectively; not to mention the possible effects of weather; and other environmental factors that can have either a positive or negative impact on our breathing.

As an example, think about how your body reacts when you step outside on a cold winter day as opposed to when it's hot and humid; or how you feel after indulging in a big meal or having a few too many cocktails. Using temperature as an example, we know that our body functions best at a temperature of 98.6 degrees Fahrenheit. This is the reason why we sweat in the summer and shiver in the winter as our body attempts to cool and warm itself, respectively.

Breathing is Multi-Systemic

Breathing is also *multi-systemic*. Contrary to what many people believe, breathing is not just a function of the lungs and the respiratory system alone. In fact, multiple systems contribute to the act of breathing including the following:

- Neurologic system (brain, spinal cord, and nerves)
- Cardiovascular system (heart and circulation)
- Musculoskeletal system (muscles, bones, joints)
- Endocrine system (glands and hormones)
- Gastrointestinal system (digestion and the digestive tract)
- Hematopoietic System (blood and the production of blood cells)

While each system is specialized to perform a different function or set of functions, they are also interconnected, working together; constantly monitoring and adapting to changes in the internal and external environment to establish a physiologic state of balance known as *equilibrium*.

The net impact of each system will vary depending on the individual, and their condition and *co-morbidities*, i.e., other medical issues. Other systems can and will be involved on an individual, case-by-case basis. Therefore, it is essential that you, along with your doctor, investigate and explore all the factors that *could* potentially be contributing to your shortness of breath.

The Respiratory System

The primary functions of the *respiratory system* are to deliver oxygen (O2) to the body and remove carbon dioxide (CO2) and other waste products of metabolism. At the most basic level, when you take a breath, O2 molecules enter the lungs and cross into the bloodstream. This *"oxygenated"* blood is then transported to the heart, where it is pumped to every cell and organ of the body for use as fuel during metabolism.

CO2 and other metabolic waste products cross from the cells and organs of the body into the bloodstream. This *"deoxygenated"* blood is then transported back to the heart, where it is pumped to the lungs, where CO2 is expelled during exhalation.

Inhalation

Inhalation is an *active* process, meaning that it requires the active muscular contraction of the *diaphragm,* the *primary muscle of inspiration* (and the *intercostal* muscles) for it to occur. For us to take a breath, the brain sends a signal down the spinal cord to the phrenic nerve. When the *phrenic nerve* innervates (i.e., sends an impulse to) the diaphragm, it contracts downward, creating a *negative pressure* in the *thoracic cavity.* It is this negative pressure that causes the lungs to inflate, filling up with air.

When breathing demands increase—as in the case of physical activity or exertion, or in the context of respiratory disease, your body can call on the *accessory muscles,* which include the muscles of the neck, back, and chest, among others, to assist with ventilation.

People with *restrictive lung diseases,* such as *Pulmonary Fibrosis* and other ILD's, typically have a difficult time with the *inhalation* phase of breathing due to increased stiffness of the lungs. As a result, they must generate significantly greater force in the respiratory muscles to overcome the increased lung resistance.

People with restrictive lung disease often take shallow breaths with less air in each inhalation. As a result, they are forced to breathe more rapidly to keep up with the body's ventilation and respiration demands. This contrasts with people who have *obstructive lung diseases (like COPD or Asthma),* who have difficulty in expelling air *out* of the lungs.

Exhalation

During quiet breathing, exhalation is a mostly passive process, relying on relaxation of the respiratory muscles, and the natural elastic recoil of the lungs, which causes them to deflate and expel air. Exhalation can also become an active process when the expiratory muscles, particularly the abdominals, contract to actively force air out of the lungs. This *forced exhalation* can be done voluntarily or involuntarily and can occur during strenuous (or not so strenuous) activity, particularly in cases of impaired lung function.

People with obstructive lung diseases, such as COPD have a difficult time getting air *out* of the lungs during exhalation. This can be caused by several factors including airway inflammation, mucus or spasm in the airways, a decrease in the natural recoil in the lungs or the destruction of the small airways and alveoli. This contrasts with people with restrictive disease, who have *increased* recoil.

Ventilation and Respiration

The mechanical act of moving air in and out of the lungs, i.e., inhalation and exhalation, is called *ventilation*. Ventilation is an *active* process, meaning that it requires the contraction and relaxation of the respiratory muscles, for it to occur.

The chemical exchange of oxygen (O_2) and carbon dioxide (CO_2) between the external environment and the cells of the body is called *respiration* or *gas exchange*. Respiration is a passive process and occurs constantly, regardless of muscle activity or phase of ventilation. In other words, it occurs at the cellular level, during both inhalation and exhalation, as well as during any pauses in between.

While there are many factors involved in how well your body uses oxygen, its overall efficiency is based upon three main factors:

1. How effectively your lungs move air in and out
2. How effectively your heart pumps blood
3. How efficiently your muscles utilize oxygen

If there is a problem in any one of these areas, your body will not be as efficient at using oxygen and you will be shorter of breath. For example, if you have a chronic respiratory disease, your lungs will not move air in and out as effectively. If you've had a *myocardial infarction* (heart attack), your heart will not pump blood as effectively. If you lead a sedentary lifestyle, then your muscles will not utilize oxygen as effectively.

If you have problems in more than one area (which is not uncommon), your breathing (and other issues) can multiply. As an example, if you have both heart and lung disease, you will likely have significantly more difficulty than if you had either one alone.

Here is the good news, though, and again, I am completely biased. *But*...in our experience, we have found that the *right* combination and type of exercise and breathing techniques can *significantly* improve the effectiveness of the respiratory, cardiovascular, and muscular systems, thereby improving your body's overall efficiency at using oxygen.

Chapter 5:

Better Breathing Techniques by Noah Greenspan, PT, DPT, CCS, EMT-B

By a landslide, the chief complaint that I hear most often from patients is shortness of breath. For that reason, we have decided to place this chapter early in the book because we truly believe that these breathing techniques can have a *major* impact on your life in a relatively short amount of time, giving you greater control over your breathing, reducing your anxiety, and allowing you to participate in more of the activities that you want to; in other words, living your life.

As I've already mentioned, for most people, shortness of breath usually begins at high levels of activity such as stair-climbing or walking uphill. To make matters worse, human nature is such that we find every reason under the sun to avoid the activity or activities that cause us shortness of breath. It's like the old joke where a patient says: "Doc, it hurts when I do this," and the doctor replies: "well, don't do that." Similarly, if you get short of breath when you "do that," odds are you aren't going to "do that" very often.

The problem is that once you start eliminating those higher-level activities, all the muscles you use to climb stairs, walk uphill or run for a bus become deconditioned and when muscles become deconditioned, they become less efficient at utilizing oxygen and you then become shorter of breath at lower levels of activity. When it comes to SOB, deconditioning is the number one enemy, and our number one goal is to help you break this *dyspnea cycle*.

It can be very easy to get caught in the dyspnea cycle of shortness of breath and inactivity, and very difficult to get out. Too often, people avoid the activities that cause them shortness of breath, and for good reason. They're terrified! However, in many cases, this inactivity can become more debilitating than their original respiratory impairment. For example, someone stops taking the subway because climbing subway stairs makes them short of breath. Then, they find ways to avoid the blocks with inclines, and before they know it, even walking on flat surfaces causes them to gasp for air.

People find all kinds of reasons to stop doing the things that cause them discomfort. For many people, the biggest one is fear. For others, it's their doctor or other health care professionals telling them to "take it easy." Still, others are waiting until they feel better before resuming their normal activities or beginning a new program. However, without some form of action or intervention, that day may never come. In fact, the longer you do nothing, the more difficult it will be, the longer it will take and the less likely it will be that you get moving again.

Keep in mind that increased shortness of breath does not necessarily indicate that your lung function has gotten worse. It is completely possible that your breathing difficulty has gotten worse solely due to inactivity or any one of a thousand other explanations other than a decline in pulmonary function. So, don't throw in the towel just yet.

The good news is that by gaining greater control of your breathing—first, when you are at rest, then during activity, and finally, when you are in distress—your breathing can improve and so can your life.

Here is some more good news. In the same way that your condition can spiral downwards under the *wrong* conditions, it can also spiral upwards under the *right* conditions, by implementing positive lifestyle changes. I prefer to use the term "life changes," because the term "lifestyle changes" sounds like we'll no longer be "wintering in Miami" or "summering in the Hamptons." And as I've said many times before: "if you want to change your life, you have to change your life."

In the same way that you have gradually eliminated activities that have become difficult for you, you can gradually begin to build those activities back into your daily routine. Again, I'm not saying it will be easy. *Again*, it won't. However, you're worth the effort of trying, and there are strategies and techniques that can help you get moving again. These include things like taking your medications properly, learning more effective breathing techniques, exercising, eating better, learning how to manage your stress and anxiety, and taking steps to *prevent* infection.

Before we go any further, let me be clear about one thing. I am not in any way trying to minimize or downplay the role of the respiratory system in shortness of breath. After all, the cardiopulmonary system is my favorite biological system for a reason. I am also not suggesting that by incorporating these breathing techniques, or by switching from white bread to wheat that all your breathing problems will go away overnight. They won't. What I *am* saying is that with a little bit of knowledge and effort, you *can* generate positive changes in your body and your life.

This chapter provides you with practical information and simple instructions on how you can regain control of your breathing. My mentor Dr. Pineda used to say: "Some people wait for things to happen; some people make things happen and some people say, 'what happened'?" Well, get ready, my friends because we are about to make things happen.

Now, take a deep breath and let's begin.

The Breathing Techniques: Breaking the Cycle

The first step in breaking the dyspnea cycle is to learn the *controlled breathing techniques (CBT)* that will help you better manage your SOB, or ideally, prevent it in the first place. These include *Pursed Lip Breathing (PLB), Diaphragmatic Breathing (aka abdominal or belly breathing)* and *Paced Breathing*. Although initially, these techniques need to be practiced as separate entities, when I mention controlled breathing techniques or simply, "the breathing", I am referring to using a combination of all three techniques together.

I will also teach you what we commonly refer to as *Recovery from Shortness of Breath*. Based upon my experience, the question that patients want answered first and foremost, is what to do when you simply cannot catch your breath. By far, this is the scenario that people fear most and what I believe prevents many people from being able to break the dyspnea cycle. After all, few things in life are scarier than not being able to breathe or as the American Lung Association says: "if you can't breathe, nothing else matters."

Again, please remember that no single breathing technique will work best for every person in all situations. Also, don't expect *anything* to work immediately or even very quickly. It will take a little time for you to start seeing progress, as well as some personal trial and error. After all, you didn't get into this hole overnight. You aren't getting out overnight either. If pressed for an answer, I would estimate that most people start to feel at least *slightly* better after approximately 3-4 weeks.

Don't let that discourage you. In fact, I think it should be encouraging. My recommendation would be to try out the techniques—all of them—and practice them. And by practice them, I don't mean try them once or twice and pray for a miracle. Try each of them under different circumstances and conditions. Give each technique several chances to work so you really have an opportunity to evaluate what works for you and what doesn't. Trust me. This will be a worthwhile investment of your time and effort. So, please be patient with the techniques and yourself.

Controlled Breathing Techniques

If you have seen any of the UPW webinars or previously participated in a pulmonary rehabilitation program, you may be familiar with some or even all "the breathing" techniques. Again, please understand that while I will describe each technique separately and you will practice each of them individually, you will use all three in concert during exercise and activity. So, when I say, do "the breathing", I am referring to all three of these techniques used together for maximum effectiveness.

Before we begin, take a moment to observe your "normal" breathing pattern. Are your respirations rapid and shallow or slow and deep? Do you breathe using your abdomen or are you relying on the *accessory muscles* of your upper chest, shoulders, back and neck? By first observing your current breathing pattern, you will start to become more conscious of which muscles and which breathing techniques are working effectively and where you might need to make some changes.

OK. Here it is. The moment you've all been waiting for—time to discuss the actual techniques that will help you break this vicious cycle of SOB and inactivity.

Pursed-Lip Breathing (Pursed-Lip Exhalation)

Pursed-lip breathing (PLB) can help you prolong exhalation, slow down your breathing, and help keep your airways open—all good things. PLB can be used in any position and regardless of whether you breathe in through your nose or mouth. In fact, as an exercise, I would suggest that you practice performing pursed-lip exhalations, breathing in through both your nose AND your mouth (at different times, of course). For the purposes of this exercise, don't worry so much about the timing (yet). Instead, just take note of what it feels like to exhale through pursed lips.

As you breathe in, imagine "smelling the flowers" and as you breathe out through pursed lips, imagine "cooling the soup on a spoon." And please don't blow your soup clear across the room. Just try to cool it off a little. People often use the suggestion, "blow out the candles." However, this is the *opposite* of what we want since the goal of all the controlled breathing techniques will almost always be relaxed, easy breathing.

As you breathe in, you should feel your abdomen rise. As you breathe out, you should feel your abdomen fall, all the while, keeping your upper chest, shoulders, back and neck muscles as quiet (still) and relaxed as possible. Try a few cycles and observe the changes in your body. Is your breathing becoming slower and deeper? Are you becoming more relaxed? *If yes, you are doing it right.*

To practice pursed-lip exhalations while breathing *in through the nose*:

1. Sit or recline comfortably in a chair.
2. Relax your upper chest, shoulders, back and neck muscles.
3. Inhale slowly through your nose.
4. Exhale slowly through pursed lips.
5. Repeat

When breathing in through your mouth, imagine sipping slowly through a straw as you breathe in and cooling your soup as you breathe out. Again, as you breathe in, you should feel your abdomen rise. As you breathe out, you should feel your abdomen fall, all the while, keeping your upper chest, shoulders, back and neck muscles as quiet as possible.

To practice pursed-lip exhalations while breathing *in through the mouth*:

1. Sit or recline comfortably in a chair.
2. Relax your upper chest, shoulders, back and neck muscles.
3. Inhale slowly through your mouth.
4. Exhale slowly through pursed lips.
5. Repeat

Diaphragmatic, Abdominal or Belly, Breathing

As I mentioned before, the diaphragm is the primary muscle of *inspiration*. If you've ever watched a baby breathe, you may have noticed that their belly moves in and out with every breath. In other words, they are breathing diaphragmatically. The *diaphragm* is a big, strong muscle, making *diaphragmatic breathing* the most efficient and effective way of moving air in and out of the lungs. In fact, we should all breathe diaphragmatically, whether we have a respiratory illness or not.

This allows the diaphragm to function most effectively, giving it the greatest mechanical advantage while trying to quiet the accessory or secondary muscles of ventilation: those of the upper chest, shoulders, back, and neck. To be clear, it is impossible for us to take a breath without contraction of the diaphragm, so technically, all breathing is diaphragmatic breathing. However, since most of us have become *most* familiar with the use of the term "diaphragmatic breathing," I will use this term for consistency. As they say, you can't fight City Hall. Just keep in mind that when we use the term "diaphragmatic breathing," we are really referring to abdominal or belly breathing.

As we get older, factors such as illness, injury, emotional and even social factors can impact our breathing, causing us to become "diaphragmatically incorrect". That was a political joke. As an example, stress and anxiety can cause us to breathe less effectively, taking rapid, shallow breaths and using our upper chest muscles, as opposed to using the diaphragm most effectively. Other factors like respiratory muscle weakness, respiratory diseases, obesity or anorexia; and deconditioning can also impair our breathing, making us work harder with each breath. As a result, many of us have developed some very poor breathing habits. If this sounds like you, it will take a little time and effort to unlearn these habits, but it can be done.

To practice diaphragmatic breathing:

1. Sit or recline comfortably in a chair.
2. Relax your upper chest, shoulders, back and neck muscles.

3. Inhale slowly through your nose. As you inhale, your abdomen should rise as your lungs fill up with air, while keeping your upper chest as still as possible.
4. Exhale slowly through pursed lips (PLB). As you do this, your abdomen should fall.
5. Repeat

Paced Breathing

At this time, we will address the issue of supply and demand by combining the two previously mentioned techniques, *pursed lip breathing* and *diaphragmatic breathing,* in a coordinated effort, called *Paced Breathing.*

As you increase your activity level, your body requires a greater supply of *oxygen* (air) to meet the greater demand of the activity. Therefore, it will be to your advantage to incorporate breathing techniques that allow for the greatest amount of flow, while at the same time, minimizing airway obstruction and air trapping. Again, I would recommend trying them all to figure out which ones will become your "go to" techniques.

The most used pacing pattern is to exhale for twice as long as you inhale. For example, try breathing in through your nose for a count of two and exhaling through pursed lips for a count of four (or 3:6, or 4:8). Breathing in for a count of one and out for two is usually too short and not often effective for most people although sometimes there's no alternative. People with restrictive lung diseases like PF often have two issues with this pattern. They may find it difficult to breathe in for 2 or longer and they may find it difficult to maintain a prolonged exhalation.

If you have a *restrictive* disease, I will still suggest starting with in for 2 and out for 4 (or in for 3 and out for 6 or in for 4 and out for 8). If those don't work, I would suggest trying to shorten the exhalation so I would try in for 2 out for 3, or in for 3 and out for 5.

To practice paced breathing:

1. Sit comfortably on a chair.
2. Relax your upper chest, shoulders, back and neck muscles.
3. Inhale slowly through your nose for a count of 2.
4. Exhale slowly through pursed lips for a count of 4.
5. Repeat

As you become more comfortable with these techniques, start to utilize paced breathing during your everyday activities, while trying to keep your focus on both pursed-lip and diaphragmatic breathing. Don't worry if you don't get it at first. Learning these strategies is a process and will take some time. To be clear, for most people, this is not a natural breathing pattern so don't expect it to become automatic. It won't.

When you use all three techniques together – *diaphragmatic, pursed–lip,* and *paced breathing,* you are doing "*the breathing,*" which I will discuss further in the chapter on activities of daily living (ADL).

Recovery from Shortness of Breath

Finally, finally, let's discuss a topic called *Recovery from Shortness of Breath*. Now, *please...do not* wait until you are in what I refer to as a *"Code Red" situation* before trying to remember these techniques. In fact, the time to begin this training and practice these techniques is when you are comfortable and relaxed (i.e., *now*).

Most of you know this feeling all too well. You can't breathe. Your chest feels tight, and you are suddenly aware of every heartbeat. And as if that's not enough, panic sets in! I can assure you that panic will not help *any* situation. In fact, panic will cause you to breathe even faster and shallower, making the situation worse. Sound familiar? This *"fight or flight"* response can trigger a whole cascade of physiologic responses, few of which will be helpful to you.

Let's use stair climbing as an example. Sometimes, just the thought of walking up a flight of stairs is enough to increase your anxiety and shortness of breath. As you start to climb, you can feel your breathing becoming more labored and it feels as though your heart is beating out of your chest. You wonder if you might pass out or have a heart attack. Some of you may even think you're going to die.

By this point, you don't know who or what is in control. Is it the shortness of breath? Is it the chest tightness? Maybe it's the anxiety. The only thing you know for sure is that it's not you. This is it!

CODE RED! Is it any wonder that people choose to avoid activities that cause *this*? So, what can you do about it?

There are specific actions you can take that will help you to prevent, relieve and recover from shortness of breath. The first (and most important) one is to stop whatever you're doing; second, talk to yourself; third, get into the right position; fourth, start the breathing and fifth, re-assess your situation.

Now, ideally, you would have begun your controlled breathing techniques long before you ever got to this point, but now is not the time for "I told you so."

These are the steps for recovery from shortness of breath:

1. Stop!

First and foremost, stop whatever you're doing that got you in trouble. If it is walking, stop walking. If it is stair climbing, stop climbing. It is highly unlikely that you will be able to regain control of your breathing while continuing the activity that made you short of breath in the first place. Your immediate goal is to put out the fire and at this moment, your supply of air is not meeting the demand of the activity. Therefore, you need to decrease or eliminate the demand by immediately stopping whatever it is you're doing at the time.

2.   Talk to yourself.

I'm not talking about some crazy "One Flew Over the Cuckoo's Nest" type of conversation or that long string of expletives that might run through your mind at a time like this. Instead, now is the time to remind yourself that you do know what to do and that you have some tools in your arsenal that will help you get out of this jam.

My suggestion of what you might say to remind yourself that you know what to do, would be something original, like "*I know what to do.*" You can also use "*relax,*" "*I am OK,*" "*calm down,*" or whatever phrase or mantra you find most helpful. *And…*the good news is that once you finish this chapter, you *will* know what to do. Then it's a matter of practicing the techniques and getting better at them so that you can start to nip that snowball effect in the bud or ideally, avoid it altogether.

Don't get me wrong. Self-talk is not a magic trick that instantly reverses your shortness of breath. Instead, it's a personal call to action, reminding you that you *can* help yourself as opposed to being a passive recipient of all the wonderful gifts that living with a pulmonary disease keeps on giving (sarcasm intended). Given the choice, I will always choose to act rather than to wait and see what happens.

This is the mindset that you need to adopt when you start to feel short of breath. Remind yourself that you know what to do. Be present. Be in the moment. Be confident. If not, fake it 'til you make it. And if that doesn't work, you might benefit from enrolling in a formal pulmonary rehabilitation program where qualified medical professionals will monitor you and you can develop the skills and confidence you need.

3.   Assume the Position!

Body position can play a tremendous role in how well or how poorly you breathe. There are certain positions that will give you the greatest chance of catching your breath by allowing your diaphragm and your lungs to work more effectively, while others will make breathing more difficult or impossible, like bending over to tie your shoes. By knowing these positions and how to utilize them to your advantage, you will have a much greater chance of minimizing your shortness of breath.

The first part of the position is to bend over. The second part is to fix your upper extremities. In other words, lean forward on your arms.

If you are standing, there are a couple of different ways you can do this. One is by leaning your back against a wall or other stable surface, bending forward at the waist, and placing your hands on your thighs or knees, putting the weight through your arms.

Another option is to lean forward against a wall, table, or other stable surface, bending forward at the waist, and placing your hands or elbows and forearms on the wall or table, again, putting the weight through your arms.

If you are sitting, spread your legs wide apart; bend forward at the waist, and place your elbows and forearms on your thighs or knees, again, putting the weight through your arms.

These positions are effective because they allow the abdominal contents to drop forward, clearing the way for the diaphragm to contract downward more easily. In doing so, the diaphragm, lungs and entire body have the greatest mechanical advantage for breathing, allowing you to move air in and out most freely and effectively.

4. **Begin the Controlled Breathing Techniques.**

By this point in your "Code Red" situation (after a brief conversation with yourself), you should already have stopped what you were doing and assumed one of the recovery positions. Now, begin the controlled breathing techniques. Breathe in through your nose and out through pursed lips, breathing in for a count of 2 and out for a count of 4 (or whichever count works best for you), until you fully regain control of your breathing.

5.   **Reassess and Adapt.**

After you have calmed down and regained control of your breathing, re-assess the situation and if necessary, modify the activity that caused your shortness of breath in the first place. Sometimes this can be as simple as walking more slowly or starting the breathing techniques *before* you're in trouble.

To practice recovery from SOB:

1.   Stop what you are doing.
2.   Talk to yourself, reminding yourself that you know what to do.
3.   Assume the position.
4.   Begin the controlled breathing techniques.
5.   Reassess and adapt.

And there you have it. That's "the breathing." Remember that no single breathing technique will work best for everyone. Therefore, every technique will require some trial and error to figure out which ones are most effective *for you*. Breathe easy, my friends!

Chapter 6:

Activities of Daily Living

Supply and Demand

Over the course of any given day, some activities will naturally be more demanding than others. As an example, stair climbing is one of the more challenging activities that most of us encounter in our everyday lives and requires significantly greater effort than walking uphill. Walking uphill requires significantly greater effort than walking on a flat surface and each of those activities requires significantly greater effort than sitting on the couch watching TV or sipping a martini; or sitting on the couch watching TV *and* sipping a martini (or sitting on a martini watching the couch).

In addition to the activity itself, we must also consider the conditions under which each activity takes place. Sticking with our stair-climbing example, most people find it much more taxing to walk up a flight of stairs on a hot, humid day or after indulging in a big meal as compared to when weather conditions are more favorable; or shortly after you've taken your rescue inhaler. In addition, various other factors can also negatively impact your breathing, such as anxiety, indoor and outdoor air pollution; or having a cold, flu, or pulmonary exacerbation, among many, many others. As I say over and over (and over) again, breathing is multi-factorial.

With this concept in mind, it can be helpful to observe the activities that cause you the most difficulty, as well as the related demands they put upon your respiratory, cardiovascular, muscular, and skeletal systems...*and your emotional mind*. It is also helpful to understand that there are ways we can increase the supply side of the equation as well, using various strategies and techniques. The purpose of this chapter is to help you evaluate your own activities of daily living (ADL) and to understand how these various factors affect you, as well as what you can do to stack the odds in your favor.

Keep in mind that you won't always be able to change the physical requirements of an activity, and even more rarely will you be able to change the external environment. However, once you become attuned to which factors have the greatest impact on your performance, both positive and negative, you will be able to incorporate practices such as controlled breathing techniques, optimal timing of your medications, and using your supplemental oxygen to your greatest advantage; in addition to avoiding respiratory triggers such as pollution, temperature, and weather extremes; and allergens.

Just because an activity makes you uncomfortable doesn't necessarily mean that it must be avoided completely, and in many cases, quite the opposite is true. It shouldn't be. Remember that your body gets good at what you ask it (or don't ask it) to do, and over time, gradually increasing these difficult activities can improve your ability. However, to improve your performance, you will need to find ways to become more efficient and effective at performing these activities, so you can once again regain control of your breathing and your life; in other words, you will need to work smarter, not harder. Let's look at some of the factors that play a role in breathing and activity.

NOTE: As always, please clear any intended lifestyle changes with your physician.

Aerobic Capacity

Aerobic capacity refers to the efficiency and effectiveness with which your body utilizes oxygen to support physiologic activity. This is largely based on three main factors.

- How effectively your lungs move air in and out
- How effectively your heart pumps blood
- How efficiently your skeletal muscles utilize oxygen

As I have mentioned previously, a problem in any one of these areas can impact your performance. However, if you have problems in more than one area, such as heart *and* lung disease, you will likely have significantly greater difficulty than either one alone.

Air Supply and Oxygen Demand: Respiratory Mechanics and Metabolism

For us to take a breath, the brain sends a signal down the spinal cord to the phrenic nerve, which innervates the diaphragm, activating it to contract downward. This downward contraction creates

a negative pressure in the thoracic cavity, causing the lungs to fill
with air.

People with restrictive lung diseases like PF and other ILD's typically have difficulty with the *inhalation phase,* i.e., moving air
in. However, inhalation and exhalation are like Yin and Yang,
meaning that if you have difficulty with one phase, it will also
affect the other, with the result being the same; shortness of breath,
decreased muscle strength and decreased activity tolerance. This
explains why you can be short of breath even in the presence of
normal or even high oxygen content in the blood, i.e., saturation.

In the case of a strictly mechanical problem, supplemental oxygen
will not help you. Instead, the solution lies in performing the
controlled breathing techniques, clearing your secretions, and
taking your rescue inhaler (if you have one), in the short term; and
gradual, but progressive exercise, over the long term. Respiratory
mechanics *can* affect metabolism and oxygen saturation. In the
case where your shortness of breath *is* accompanied by a decrease
in oxygen saturation, you *will* benefit from supplemental oxygen,
adjusting or *titrating* the amount based upon your pulse oximeter
readings. In fact, if your oxygen saturation falls below 90%, I would
strongly recommend speaking with your doctor about supplemental oxygen use. We will discuss this in greater detail in the next
chapter on oxygen.

Finally, on the flip side, there are a group of people who are hypoxic,
yet do not feel particularly breathless. This often occurs in people
who have been living with a respiratory disease for a long period
of time as they have become desensitized to their dyspnea. In this

situation, you should also be using supplemental oxygen; adjusting or *titrating* the amount based upon your oximeter readings. If your oxygen saturation is in the nineties, preferably 93% plus, you're good. If your saturation is below 90%, turn up the oxygen or switch from a cannula to a mask. This is what I mean when I talk about "relying on your instruments," as opposed to adjusting based solely on how you are feeling at that moment.

Energy Cost and Metabolic Equivalents

MET level, or metabolic equivalents are a measurement of physiologic workload or exercise tolerance, in other words, the energy cost of the activity. Every activity comes with its own metabolic price tag, which corresponds to the amount of oxygen consumed. Activities that are less than three METs are considered light. Activities between three and six METs are considered moderate and activities that are six METs or greater are considered heavy or vigorous activity.

Below are some sample activities and their corresponding MET level. Please keep in mind that these are *rough* estimates, and *many* factors can affect individual MET level.

- 1 MET: energy expenditure at rest, lying in bed
- 1.0 to 1.9 METs: eating, grooming, shaving (sitting), writing
- 2.0 to 2.9 METs: cooking, making the bed, showering (warm), dressing (sitting)

- 3.0 to 3.9 METs: vacuuming, showering (warm), dressing (standing), walk 3 mph
- 4.0 to 4.9 METs: gardening, swimming,
- 5.0 to 5.9 METs: Showering (hot, standing)
- 6.0 to 6.9 METs: stair climbing (down)

Activities of Daily Living

When I polled the members of our *Ultimate Pulmonary Wellness Facebook Group*, the three activities that were reported to be most difficult were stair climbing, walking uphill, and walking quickly... *by a landslide.* As I mentioned at the beginning of this chapter, walking up a flight of stairs requires significantly more effort than walking on an incline i.e., uphill; and walking uphill, sometimes even if it's only a slight incline, requires significantly more effort than walking on flat ground.

Walking

Like breathing itself, locomotion in all its forms is a multi-factorial process that both *affects* and is *affected by* many variables. Walking increases your body's demand for both air (mechanical) and oxygen (metabolic). For that reason, it is important for us to have strategies at our disposal to either reduce the energy demands of the activity or to increase the supply of air and oxygen.

Other factors to consider include: the longer and steeper the stairs, the greater the metabolic demand. The faster you walk, the greater the demand. Carrying something while you walk or walking and talking will also increase the demand; and just in case you're sensing a theme here, the more challenging the activity, the greater the demand. Emotional factors like anxiety can also play a role; both affecting and being affected by breathing and activity, decreasing the supply of air *and* increasing the metabolic demand.

Here are some techniques you can incorporate when you're walking:

Practice "the Breathing."

When it comes to walking, by far, the greatest tools you have are your controlled breathing techniques. Diaphragmatic, pursed lip and paced breathing will give you greater breath control, allowing you to walk more. Time your breathing with your walking, with each step being one count. Try breathing in for two steps and out for four steps or whichever pattern you find most beneficial. The same is true for stair climbing, using each step as a count of one. If this is too vigorous, you can modify the activity even further. Instead of one step for each count, breathe in while standing still and exhale as you start to climb again.

Pace Yourself!

Walk as slowly as you need to maintain control of your breathing. Walking at a slower pace will reduce the metabolic demand of the activity. If you're still having trouble maintaining control of your breathing, stop walking and perform the techniques for *recovery from shortness of breath*. Once you have regained control of your breathing, you can start walking again...*slowly*.

Take your "rescue" medication before exercise or activity.

Taking your rescue medication; typically, a short-acting bronchodilator; increases the supply of air and oxygen by opening the airways, allowing you to take a deeper breath. Taking it approximately 15 minutes before exercise should help you have your best workout. One point that you may ask your doctor about is this. Although bronchodilators do not typically demonstrate a benefit to patients with restrictive lung disease when you take a pulmonary function test (PFT), many anecdotally report symptomatic relief from them. Again, you can ask your doctor if he, she, or they think it might be worth a try.

Increase your supplemental oxygen as necessary.

If your oxygen saturation drops below 90%, increase the liter flow or switch to a mask. Again, we will discuss this further in the next chapter.

Use a shopping cart or rolling walker.

Using a shopping cart or rolling walker closes the chain, improving respiratory mechanics; not only decreasing the metabolic demand of the activity, but also increasing the supply of air and oxygen.

Relax!!!

I realize that this is usually easier said than done. However, *try* to prepare yourself mentally and emotionally for the activity. As an example, before you start up a flight of stairs, take a moment or two to compose yourself and start your controlled breathing techniques proactively, *before* starting up the stairs.

Shhh...

Many people find walking and talking difficult. Talking is essentially continuous exhaling, which will quickly reduce your available supply of air. Pace your breathing so that you are speaking during what would normally be the exhalation phase, and by taking slow, deep breaths in between speaking, while the other person is talking. Think of it as an opportunity to work on your listening skills.

Lifting and Carrying

Lifting and carrying, especially heavy objects, can significantly impair your breathing from both a supply and demand perspective. First, lifting and carrying will increase the metabolic demand to varying degrees, depending upon the load. As the load increases, so will the metabolic demand. In addition, lifting and carrying can also decrease supply. Imagine carrying a paper bag of groceries across your chest in front of you. This compresses the thorax, mechanically preventing you from taking a deep breath.

Now think about carrying two plastic bags, one in each hand. This load pulls down on the thorax and the ribcage, increasing the amount of resistance required by the diaphragm to elevate the ribcage, again, preventing you from taking a deep breath. Again, the same factors, including walking on a flat surface, walking on an incline, and climbing stairs, will further increase the metabolic requirements.

Bending and Reaching

Bending and reaching compress your thoracic and abdominal cavities like an accordion, increasing the pressures against which, the diaphragm must contract, preventing you from taking a deep breath. There is further compression of the thorax, preventing you from taking a deep breath, and preventing the lungs from filling with air.

Another task people regularly report difficulty with is bending down to tie their shoes. This is due to thoracic and abdominal compression. Instead of trying to breathe while you are down there, prepare yourself by taking a deep breath in before you bend and slowly and gently exhale through pursed lips as you bend down and tie your shoe. As you start to run short on air, rise again as you take a deep inhalation. Then exhale through pursed lips as you bend over to tie the other shoe.

Showering and Bathing

Many people find showering and bathing extremely difficult. For both activities, there are *many* factors—almost like an "all of the above" situation. Increased humidity in the bathroom due to the hot water and steam can make you work harder to move air in *and* out. Think of inhaling and exhaling that thick air as being like drinking a milkshake through a narrow straw as compared to plain water. Instead of hot, use lukewarm or tepid water and leave the bathroom door either cracked or completely open.

Another issue has to do with the use of the upper extremities to wash; especially overhead as you do when you wash your hair. Overhead activity puts the diaphragm and the respiratory muscles at a very poor mechanical advantage, significantly increasing your shortness of breath. To decrease the work of breathing as well as the overall metabolic demand of showering, I would suggest using a shower chair or bench, as well as a hand-held shower. This will allow you to relax and focus on your breathing as you sit and wash your body, as opposed to constantly worrying about shortness of breath or worse, slipping and falling. And while we're on the subject, let me tell you that those hand-held showers are *delightful*, and throw your cannula over the top of the shower and turn your oxygen up as high as you need to.

Dressing

Getting dressed goes hand in hand with bathing. For many of the same reasons that bathing is difficult, drying yourself off and dressing can be equally, if not more difficult. Again, overhead, open chain movements like toweling dry or putting on a shirt put the diaphragm at a mechanical disadvantage. Try using terrycloth or microfiber towel or bathrobe to do the drying for you, while you sit and catch your breath.

As you are getting dressed, use your controlled breathing techniques, coordinating movement with exhalation and inhaling in between. As an example, inhale for a count of two. Exhale for a count of four as you put one arm in the sleeve. Inhale for a count of two. Exhale as you put your other arm in the other sleeve. The same principles apply to pants, socks, shoes, etc.

Cleaning and Housework

Chores like laundry (bending, lifting, carrying, reaching); vacu-uming (bending, pushing, pulling, reaching); and making the bed (bending, pulling, reaching), are also difficult for people with respiratory problems due to the increased physical and metabolic demands, positioning, and many other challenges. Add to these issues, the potential for exposure to unhealthy environmental and chemical triggers that can add insult (and inflammation) to injury. Tasks like dusting, vacuuming, sweeping, mopping, etcet-era, etcetera expose us to all kinds of potential bacteria, viruses, allergens, and other respiratory triggers in the form of dust, debris, mold, insects and animals, and their excrement; as well as the cleaning supplies themselves, among others. Any of these factors can quickly trigger the inflammatory response, constricting the airways and increasing the production of mucus, and the work of breathing. They can also make us sick. If in doubt, please don't do it yourself. At a minimum, wear a mask, ventilate the room, use an air purifier, and please choose your cleaning products carefully, opting for hypo- or ideally, non-allergenic.

Sexual Activity

Although not often talked about, sex is also a big concern for many patients. Sexual activity involves an increased mechanical and metabolic demand for air, oxygen, circulation, and aerobic capacity due to the elevated workload. In addition, there are also complex emotional aspects that can contribute to the situation, for better and for worse. Sex can be a wonderful and enjoyable experience for many people, or an extremely anxiety-provoking situation for many others; especially if you are concerned about being able to breathe, in addition to enjoying yourself and pleasing your partner.

As with other activities, a little preparation beforehand will go a long way. Think about which positions will allow you to breathe more easily while decreasing the physical and emotional demands of the activity. As an example, lying on your back may decrease your demand for air and oxygen, reducing the aerobic requirements of the activity. However, you may also need to consider how your breathing will be affected by the weight of your partner. In that case, you may want to try other positions. If you need oxygen, turn it up! If you have a rescue inhaler, ask your doctor if you can use it proactively.

Now, while I'm not trying to give you the *Kama Sutra for Pulmonary Patients*, my suggestion would be for you and your partner to experiment with various positions and practices to figure out what works best *for both of you*. Although it may be uncomfortable at first, communication is key to finding strategies that meet both partners' needs. And *breathe*! Utilize all the controlled breathing techniques, before, during, and after sex. Just be sure to skip the requisite after–sex cigarette.

Energy Conservation versus Energy Maximization

At first glance, the difference between energy conservation and energy maximization seems like nitpicking or semantics. However, there are significant differences between the two ideas: with *mindset* often being a *major* factor. In my experience, "traditional" energy conservation techniques typically focus on teaching people how to modify the activity in a downward direction to accommodate the metabolic demand. Paradoxically, while this downgrade may make the activity more manageable for the moment, it will ultimately make it become more difficult over time. Remember that your body gets good at doing what you ask it to do.

Finally, while I concede that there will be times that your limitations may get the best of you, I would much rather you take the steps to up your game to meet this increased demand as opposed to automatically downgrading all your activities. I assure you that I am *not* minimizing your struggle. I *am* encouraging you *not* to sell the farm too quickly. My goal is to encourage you to keep trying, even when things get tough. Perhaps you need to work smarter, not harder.

Chapter 7:

Supplemental Oxygen by Linda Gorman

Hello. My name is Linda. I have been on supplemental oxygen for the past 8½ years, and I am always looking for, and finding better ways to improve my oxygen usage and get the most out of my oxygen and my life.

Within this chapter, I hope to provide you with the tools you need to utilize and maximize the benefits of your oxygen in your life. I'll provide you with tips for daily living that I have learned from other oxygen users, health care professionals like Dr. Noah Greenspan, *and personal experience.* These techniques have been invaluable for me, and I hope you will also find them effective and beneficial as well.

I am sure it was very difficult first hearing that you have a serious lung condition, and then that you may need supplemental oxygen. In my experience, I have found that only those of us that use oxygen truly understand what it's like. At first, it is natural that you might feel uncomfortable or self-conscious going out in public with your oxygen. This is completely understandable. However, I hope that over time, the benefits you receive and the things that you can accomplish because of your oxygen will outweigh any discomfort or embarrassment you may feel. After all, we don't think poorly of someone on crutches. Why would we think poorly of someone who uses oxygen? And ultimately, it comes down to doing what will allow *you* to live *your* best life possible. Nobody else.

Why am I being prescribed supplemental oxygen?

Interstitial lung disease causes inflammation and/or fibrosis (scarring) in the alveoli, the tiny air sacs where gas exchange occurs. This can lower your body's ability to utilize oxygen most effectively both at rest and even more significantly, during exertion.

There are several ways that oxygen saturation can be measured. The most common method is using a device called a ***pulse oximeter***. A "pulse ox" is easy to use, accurate and non-invasive. It works by placing it on your finger, ear, or forehead, and can measure both your oxygen saturation and pulse (heart rate).

You will likely find it very helpful to have your own pulse oximeter. Personally, I keep one at home, one in my purse, and one in my car and find them indispensable. I use them to monitor my oxygen saturation and heart rate at rest, during daily activity, and exercise, making any necessary adjustments to my oxygen flow to keep my saturation in the 91-93% range and my heart rate at less than 120 beats per minute. Keep in mind that everyone is different, and these parameters should be determined by your doctor as to what heart rate and oxygen ranges are acceptable and desired for you.

Normal oxygen saturation should be between 96 to 100% but ILD can diminish that significantly, particularly with activity. Generally, if your oxygen falls below 90%, supplemental oxygen is required.

A more direct (and more invasive) method is called **Arterial Blood Gas (ABG)**. In an ABG, blood is drawn from an artery, usually in the wrist. The blood is then sent through an analyzer to measure the amount of oxygen dissolved in the blood. This result is called the partial arterial oxygen pressure (PaO2) and is normally 75-100 mm Hg.

Your healthcare doctor or other health care provider should determine the amount of supplemental oxygen you need by monitoring your saturation at rest, during activity such as walking (often done during a six-minute walk test), and during sleep via an overnight oxygen study. If sleep apnea is suspected, a formal sleep study may also be in order. Ask your doctor what level of oxygen saturation they want you to maintain in various situations and then titrate your supplemental oxygen accordingly.

If you are planning to travel by plane or to an area of altitude, a high-altitude simulation test (HAST) can also be ordered to test your oxygen saturation at various altitudes to ensure that it is safe for you to travel. As a point of reference, most commercial airlines maintain a cabin pressure equal to approximately 8000 feet.

Once it is determined you need oxygen, your health care provider will write a prescription specifying the appropriate oxygen flow rate that will keep you properly "saturated." This is expressed in liters per minute, for example, 2 liters per minute (lpm) or as a numerical *setting* on a portable concentrator.

Your doctor or other health care professional (RT, RN, CPT, etc.) should also be able to refer you to an appropriate oxygen or durable medical equipment (DME) supplier and help you determine the type of equipment that will best accommodate your lifestyle. Your doctor will also be required to fill out the necessary paperwork to ensure that your oxygen is covered by your insurance.

How do I choose the right oxygen device and equipment?

Your doctor, health care provider, and oxygen supplier should all work with you to choose the oxygen system that is right for *you*; one that considers your medical condition as well as your lifestyle and activity level. The goal is to have the oxygen equipment that will be the most effective, most comfortable and that will allow you to enjoy your best life possible and the activities that are important to you.

Some of the factors to consider when choosing your equipment are:

- How much oxygen do you require?
- What is the size and layout of your home, and do you have stairs?
- How long and how often do you leave your house?
- What activities do you do while you are out?
- Your size, strength, and conditioning level
- The size and weight of the equipment
- Your personal preferences

The types of oxygen systems currently available are:

- Metal Tanks (Steel or Aluminum)
- Home (Stationary) Concentrator
- Portable Oxygen Concentrators (POC)
- Liquid Oxygen

Metal Tanks (Steel or Aluminum)

One of the most used delivery methods is compressed oxygen that comes in either a steel or aluminum tank. Tanks deliver 100% medical grade oxygen, and you control the flow using a regulator that can be either *continuous* or *pulsed* to conserve oxygen.

Obviously, the smaller and lighter the tank, the less oxygen it will hold and therefore, the less time you will have before you need to change it. Take this into consideration when you and your doctor are deciding on the best system for you. There is an app called O2toGo (https://respondo2.com/cylinder-duration/) that can help you determine how long your tank will last based upon your liter flow. I check my tank about 15-30 minutes before the end of the calculated duration to ensure I'm not running lower than expected.

Oxygen Concentrators

Oxygen concentrators draw air in from your surroundings, remove nitrogen and other gases and deliver purified oxygen to the user. They can be stationary or portable.

Home or stationary concentrators deliver oxygen continuously and operate on electricity. Stationary concentrators can supply higher liter flows (currently as high as 10 liters per minute, depending upon the unit) and they won't run out of oxygen if they are functioning properly, remain plugged in, and you don't lose power.

Because they need electricity to work, you will need to have a backup plan in case of a power outage. I live in a high fire and wind area with multiple power outages and rolling blackouts every year. For that reason, I have 3 E tanks to use as a backup. In addition, I have notified my electric company that I am on oxygen in case of outages, *and* I receive a discount to my electric bill to boot. Contact your local supplier to see what accommodations may be available to you in your area.

Portable Oxygen Concentrators (POC's) run on batteries, so they can be used anywhere, except in water and extreme temperatures. They typically come with both AC and DC chargers, that enable you to save your battery life if you are near an electrical outlet.

POC's can be continuous; pulsed, meaning that it will only deliver oxygen upon inhalation; or have both options. Due to their size and relatively limited ability to generate oxygen, POC's are not recommended for people who require more than 3 lpm of continuous flow .

Whether you are using a concentrator or tank, when you are using a device in pulsed mode, the numerical settings are *not* equal to the liters per minute (lpm) on a continuous flow device. In other words, a setting of 3 pulsed does *not* mean 3 liters per minute. To find out the actual amount being delivered; you would have to check with the individual manufacturer's specifications or another reliable source.

One of the best sources (if not the single-best source) for information on POC's is the Pulmonary Paper's annual Portable Oxygen Concentrator Guide, written by Ryan Diesem, RRT. This guide provides the most current POC descriptions and specifications in a useful chart that allows for easy comparisons between units.

Another great resource on oxygen usage is Noah Greenspan's *Oxygen Manifesto* series in the next chapter.

Liquid Oxygen

Liquid oxygen is a type of delivery system where oxygen is compressed and cooled, first below freezing, then to a liquid. Then, once it is exposed to warmer temperatures, it converts back into gas. Most liquid oxygen systems can provide a high liter flow and do not require any electricity. Liquid oxygen systems usually consist of a portable device and stationary "reservoir" unit for storage, that you then use to fill your portable device.

Unfortunately, liquid oxygen is not used much in the US, due to availability, cost, and insurance limitations. It is used more frequently in other countries like Canada and the UK. The portable unit is small and lasts much longer than the small oxygen tanks.

Interfaces and Accessories for your oxygen delivery system

Nasal Cannulas and Oxygen Tubing

A nasal cannula is the plastic tube that delivers oxygen from your oxygen device to your body via two small prongs that go just inside your nose. They are usually available in 4-foot and 7-foot lengths. You can also add extra extension tubing (usually 25 to 75 feet) so you can get around your home without moving your concentrator from room to room. There is also a swivel connector that attaches the cannula to the tubing to help eliminate kinking.

Nasal cannulas are low concentration conduits and work well with liter flows of less than 6 liters per minute (lpm). If your lpm requirement is 6 or more, you will need high flow tubing and cannulas, or if that is not sufficient to maintain your saturation, you should ask your doctor about switching to a mask, especially during periods of vigorous (and even not-so-vigorous) activity or exercise.

You may hear varying recommendations on cleaning so check with your doctor or health care professional for specifics, but in general, cannulas should be changed every week if used constantly or every 2 weeks if used for only a few hours each day. Change even more frequently (at least daily) if you are sick. Tubing should be changed every month.

Simple Face Mask

A simple facemask covers the nose and mouth. Your doctor may prescribe a facemask instead of a nasal cannula if you require a higher oxygen concentration, extra humidity or can't tolerate a nasal cannula. A simple mask should be cleaned twice a week with warm soapy water.

Non-Rebreather Mask

A non-rebreather mask also covers nose and mouth and has a plastic reservoir bag attached to the end that increases the concentration of oxygen delivered. This mask is useful for people that require a high continuous liter flow of oxygen as many with ILD do, especially during activity and exercise.

Humidifier

A humidifier is sometimes recommended for oxygen flows at 4 lpm or more. I found the humidifier helpful when the weather was dry, and I was getting nose bleeds. It also helps sinus dryness. The type of humidifier you use will depend on your type of home oxygen and how much oxygen you need. Many of the home concentrators have a built-in space for holding the humidifier bottle. This plastic bottle is connected to your tubing. It is recommended you use distilled water (not tap) and clean each time before refilling.

Equipment Maintenance

Different types of oxygen equipment have different requirements for cleaning and overall maintenance. Some tasks can be done by the patient themselves and some require professional maintenance. Please be sure to check with your company and have a clear understanding of what the requirements and recommendations are for your unit...*and then make sure you follow them.* Think of your oxygen apparatus as life support equipment and act accordingly.

One to Grow On!

Try to choose a system that can grow with you if you anticipate that your oxygen needs may increase in the future. I invested in an expensive POC that at its highest setting just met my needs. I was attracted to its light weight, but I was able to use it for less than a year. This was before I knew about any of the pulmonary Facebook support groups, so if you are thinking of purchasing a unit, ask around first.

Where do I get my oxygen equipment and how is it paid for?

Your doctor may help you select an oxygen or DME supplier. Some insurance plans may designate which company to use and may have restrictions on the types of devices you can use and the number of tanks you can have. Yes, that is complete BS that your medical decisions are made by an insurance company and not your physician! That last sentence was from Noah.

You may also have certain restrictions on changing companies or devices based on insurance requirements. Yes. That is also a bunch of BS (again, Noah)! So, in selecting a provider, be sure to talk to them about their policies and procedures so you don't inadvertently get locked into a situation or supplier that cannot or will not meet your needs.

If you travel often, you may want to select a nationwide provider since they can deliver the supplies you need to the hotel or address you will be visiting.

Most insurance policies cover supplemental oxygen when the medical necessity for oxygen is demonstrated. I have Medicare plus a Medicare supplement, and everything is covered including accessories. And again, please note that payment (and all other) rules can vary by jurisdiction and insurance carrier. In Canada, oxygen supplies are covered by Provincial health plans. So, be sure you know the rules in your area.

Safety Tips

Note: Some of these safety tips may seem obvious. However, keep in mind that if they are being included, there is a reason. Please don't become a statistic.

- Oxygen is not flammable, but it *can* act as an accelerant, causing fires to burn hotter and faster. This means, you must exercise extreme caution around open flames. If you have a gas stove, use extreme caution. Keep the flame low and keep your oxygen away from the flame.
- Don't use oil-based or petroleum products near your oxygen. This includes any creams, lotions, or other products such as vapor rubs, petroleum jelly or oil-based lotions and creams. Use water-based products instead.
- Notify your family, friends, and neighbors; as well as your local fire department, electric and phone companies that you use oxygen. This may be helpful in an emergency.
- Whether you use oxygen or not, DON'T SMOKE. If you must smoke, don't smoke while using your oxygen. Avoid others who are smoking.

- When fueling your vehicle, turn off your oxygen (and your vehicle). Or even better, have someone else pump your gas for you.
- Don't store your oxygen in a confined space, like a closet or trunk. It is recommended that you keep at least 12 inches of open space around the unit.
- Keep your liquid oxygen unit upright.
- Don't use extension cords or plug anything into the same outlet as your oxygen.
- Turn off your oxygen when not in use.
- Be careful not to trip over the tubing.

Traveling with Oxygen

Before making any travel arrangements, discuss your plans with your doctor, RT, RN, PT, family, friends, *YOUR OXYGEN/DME PROVIDER*, and anyone else that might be involved or offer any insight into the road, ocean, or sky in front of you. Make sure you are all on the same page and that you are fit to travel safely. Speak with your doctor about the following key factors:

- How long will you be travelling for?
- Will you be traveling by car, bus, RV, train, plane, boat, or cruise ship?
- What will the weather be like at your destination and are you prepared for the possibility of extreme weather and other environmental conditions such as temperature extremes (hot or cold), humidity, altitude, or air pollution?

- The names of healthcare providers, hospitals, and DME providers, both at your destination *and along the way.*
- What supplies *and what extra supplies* will you need while you're away?
- What medications, *extra medications*, and emergency medications, such as corticosteroids or antibiotics, might you need while you are away? Be sure to refill all your prescriptions before you go.
- What should you do if you have trouble breathing or other medical issues?
- What medical, insurance and personal information you should take with you and is there any type of extra insurance that you might need to purchase?
- A letter of medical necessity, authorizing you to travel with oxygen and a copy of your oxygen prescription.
- Take extra copies of all necessary documentation and keep them in a separate bag.
- If you're traveling alone, arrange to check in with a friend or family member so that person knows you're alright. If you're traveling with someone, make sure that person knows the medications you take and how to use your oxygen system. If using a POC, make sure they know how to recharge and change the batteries.

If your DME supplier is part of a national chain, ask for the contact information of a local office. Then contact that office 1 week before you arrive to make sure everything is in place or ready to go when you get there. If your DME supplier is independent, work with your contact person to find a local supplier in your destination city. If you'll be staying at a resort or hotel, let the concierge know that oxygen and oxygen supplies will be delivered to your room and that it's OK to sign for them.

NOTE: Most DME suppliers will require some time to coordinate your oxygen equipment for travel. You should provide a minimum of 2-4 weeks' notice but as a rule, the earlier the better. Share the details of your travel plans, including dates, location, and type of oxygen equipment needs, including a stationary concentrator at your destination, that will be necessary for you to travel safely.

In all these situations, it is crucial that you plan and don't just consider or assume what will happen if everything goes right. Consider what you will do if things *don't* go according to plan. I don't say this to scare you or discourage you from traveling or in any other way try to limit your plans or from living your best life possible. However, as John Steinbeck taught us: "the best laid plans of mice and men oft go astray," so plan accordingly and err on the side of overplanning than under-planning. Hope is not a strategy!

If you are traveling by Car:

- If you are using Oxygen tanks or liquid oxygen, be sure to secure them upright.
- If you are using a POC, keep your AC and DC power supplies with you. You may want to purchase a converter (DC to AC) just in case there are any problems charging

your POC from your vehicle. Also, keep your vehicle cool so your POC does not overheat.

- If you will be driving to or through high altitude areas, be aware there is less oxygen in the air at higher altitudes. So, be prepared to increase your oxygen in these areas.
- Keep emergency medications close by

NOTE: If your POC gets too hot, it will automatically shut down to prevent overheating and you will be notified of this by warning lights and/or audible alerts. This has happened to me several times on long drives. I used to place my POC on the floor of the passenger side. I now place it on the passenger seat or in the seat behind me and place a seatbelt around it. I also carry a backup M6 portable tank in case this happens.

If you are traveling by RV, keep in mind that each state has different requirements as do private campgrounds. Be sure you know what they are in advance and that they will suit your needs. This includes things like whether the campground has electricity available. Will it be enough to power all your equipment (oxygen, generator, air conditioning) and are there restrictions on the hours it can be used?

If you are traveling by Bus, be sure to contact the coach operator well in advance of your trip. Be sure that you understand their policies and procedures for traveling with oxygen. Carry a copy of your oxygen prescription and a letter from your doctor explaining why you need oxygen. If you will be using tanks, bring extras, and find out if there is a limit to the number of tanks you can bring. If you are using a POC, find out if you are allowed to recharge on the bus and try to book a seat near a 12-volt outlet. If you aren't, bring an extra battery, and know when and where the bus will stop so you can recharge. I once went on a day trip with seniors and assumed all buses had outlets. I was wrong. Luckily, I brought a spare battery.

If you are traveling by Train, be sure to contact the rail company well in advance of your trip. Be sure that you understand their policies and procedures for traveling with oxygen. As an example, in the United States, Amtrak has the following restrictions:

- If using oxygen, you can't book your trip on the Amtrak website. Instead, you must call 1-800-USA-RAIL (1-800-872-7245), and let the operator know you will be traveling with oxygen.
- If you're traveling with a POC it must be able to run on battery power for 4 hours.
- If you're traveling with liquid oxygen tanks, you're limited to two 50-pound tanks or 6 20-pound tanks.

If you are traveling by Cruise Ship, be sure to contact the cruise line well in advance of your trip. Be sure that you understand their policies and procedures for traveling with oxygen. Many cruise lines must approve your plans before you can bring oxygen equipment aboard the ship, and they may not work with DME suppliers directly. This will require you to make the arrangements with the supplier yourself to deliver the oxygen to the cruise ship.

If you are traveling by Plane, be sure to contact the airline well in advance of your trip. Be sure that you understand their policies and procedures for traveling with oxygen. Each airline is different, and many require a form to be filled out by a medical doctor before a trip, stating your specific physical condition and that you have medical approval to travel by air. Keep in mind that your oxygen needs may be different on a flight because of the difference in air pressure, even inside a pressurized cabin. If there is any doubt, ask your doctor to order a High-Altitude Simulation Test (HAST). As the name indicates, this test simulates altitude so that you will know your oxygen needs and whether you will be OK in the air. Remember, hope is not a strategy!

- Consider getting a pre-trip physical exam.
- Check with the airline before seeing your doctor to understand their requirements for flying with oxygen and/or a medical condition.
- Make sure your POC is on the Federal Aviation Agency's approved list to be taken onboard an aircraft. If it isn't, you may need to rent an approved device for your trip.
- Make sure your travel companion is familiar with your POC in case you need assistance.
- Fully charge all your batteries. Plan to have at least 2x the oxygen available than what you calculate you will need. Many airlines require you to have double the length of your entire flight duration (including layovers) in battery power for your POC. Again, this is something specific to each airline, so be sure to understand *your airline's* battery requirements in advance of your trip. Most aircrafts will not allow you to plug in your POC on board so being prepared with battery use is critical to a successful flight.

- Batteries must be kept with you in your carry-on bags. They must remain in a pressurized cabin and cannot be checked in your luggage.
- POCs are exempt from the carry-on count
- Carry an extra 3-way plug for recharging your POC in the airport. During layovers or any delays where you have access to a charging center, take advantage of it.

At the airport with POC oxygen

- Allow plenty of time for check-in
- If you get breathless when walking, arrange for help, like a wheelchair, at the airport. This should be arranged at least 48 hours before you travel. Arrange for help at any connecting airports as well.
- Inform the TSA officer that you have a POC and whether you can disconnect during the screening process. You may need to provide the letter from your doctor
- If you can disconnect, you can submit for x-ray screening or a walk-through metal detector. If you need to remain connected, your equipment will be tested for traces of explosives material.

On the plane

- You cannot sit in Exit Row seating. The FAA prohibits a person using a POC from occupying any seat in an exit row.
- The POC should be placed underneath the seat in front of you, so you or the flight attendant can see warning lights and/or hear the audible warning
- When you are on the plane, try to move every hour or so to exercise your legs.
- Drink plenty of water and non-alcoholic drinks to stay hydrated.

You have arrived

- Arrange beforehand for help, like a wheelchair to be available when you arrive
- Plan to allow time for you to rest after you arrive. You may find yourself tired.
- Have a great time and pat yourself on the back! Your future flights will be much easier now that you know the procedures

DISCLAIMER: This information is only to be used as a guide and all advice regarding travel with oxygen should be sought out and approved by a medical professional. The Federal Aviation Administration (FAA) is responsible for stipulating rules regarding the use of oxygen on board an aircraft. It is important to ensure your POC is FAA compliant and meets all the requirements to fly safely. Each physician will also require their own pre-trip health examination.

Other Tips and Tricks

- Determine how long your oxygen will last. Most patients that require more than 3 lpm at rest will need an E tank. I use 2 D tanks because they are easier for me to handle, and I put them in a rolling cart
- If you require multiple tanks, keep an extra regulator always attached to a second tank. This way, when the tank you're using gets low, you'll be ready to go *before* your oxygen runs out. It eliminates the increased anxiety (or sheer panic) of scrambling to hook up the new tank when you don't have any oxygen left.
- Have twice as many tanks as you will need. I always keep extra tanks in the car and change to a new one when I arrive at my destination, so I always have the maximum level of oxygen available.
- An *Oxymizer* or other conserving device may allow you to reduce your liter flow, thereby preserving your oxygen supply, if your oxygen demand is met adequately.
- Check with your doctor's office or rehabilitation center ahead of time, to see if they supply oxygen you can use. This will decrease the number of tanks you will need. Some of my doctors have oxygen. Others don't.

- If using POC, there may be electricity available. Ask to be seated by an outlet so you can charge while you sit, and always bring extra batteries just in case.
- If there is a long walk from the car to wherever you are going, arrange ahead of time for a wheelchair. My pulmonary rehab is quite a long walk so I do this. My pulmonary therapist wants me ready to go when I arrive.
- If you have a large POC or several tanks, arrange for assistance getting them in and out of the car.

In Conclusion

I hope you found this chapter helpful as you begin using Oxygen. It will take some adjusting to, and you will need to plan for outings. It reminds me of preparing to take my children places when they were small; lots of preparation which became easier over time. After using oxygen for a while, many people are surprised by how much better they feel and how much more active they can be.

Based on my personal experience, I recommend you become active on some Facebook groups like Ultimate Pulmonary Wellness (https://www.facebook.com/groups/UltimatePulmonaryWellness) and the Pulmonary Wellness Foundation, (https://pulmonarywellness.org), among others. These groups are invaluable and allow me to talk to others who understand what I am going through.

Chapter 8:

Oxygen Manifesto by Advice from 5 Respiratory Specialists

Written by Noah Greenspan, PT, DPT, CCS, EMT-B; Mark W. Mangus Sr., RRT, RPFT, FAARC; Ryan Diesem, RRT, RRT-NPS; Donna Frownfelter, PT, DPT, MA, CCS, RRT, FCCP; and Marion Mackles, PT, BS, LMT

Oxygen Manifesto 1: Originally printed in Pulmonary Hypertension News, March 27, 2019

One of the more hotly debated topics in the treatment of respiratory disease is supplemental oxygen use. Participants in the debate often include patients, clinicians, caretakers, suppliers, advocacy groups, and even politicians. In my experience, the information regarding when and how to use supplemental oxygen ranges in quality from the good, the bad, and in keeping with our western theme, the complete bull. It is my hope that I can help clear the air. That's my third and final western pun. Thank you very much. I'll be here all week.

Incidentally, I have previously given a webinar on this topic that you can watch HERE: https://vimeo.com/327196321

For this chapter, I have asked four respiratory and cardiopulmonary physical therapists, from whom I have learned a tremendous amount about proper oxygen supplementation, to join me in this endeavor: a man I call *Respiratory Therapist-Laureate*, Mark Mangus, *Oxygen Super-Guru* and author of the Pulmonary Paper's Portable Oxygen Concentrator (POC) Guide, Ryan Diesem, the Godmother of Chest Physical Therapy, Donna Frownfelter, and my 28-year colleague and *Mucus Buster*, Marion Mackles.

"What, Me Oxygen?" -Alfred E. Neuman

At the most basic level, your body's ability to use oxygen is based upon three main factors:

- how well your lungs move air, and consequently oxygen in and carbon dioxide out
- how well your heart pumps said oxygen-rich blood
- how efficiently your muscles utilize that oxygen

How well your body takes up and utilizes oxygen is based upon supply and demand. The good news is that all three of these factors can improve with exercise and activity and all three typically get worse with inactivity. As I say repeatedly, exercise is like pushing a car uphill. As soon as you stop pushing, you start rolling back downhill, only much more quickly. I am sure that most of us have experienced this at one time or another, so as Nike says, "Just do it!"

Why oxygen?

For people living with pulmonary fibrosis and other ILD's it is not uncommon for one or more of these above-named factors to be impaired, causing hypoxemia and hypoxia, low oxygenation in the blood and tissues.

Oxygen Assessment

How much oxygen a person has in their blood can be determined by one of two tests, either by arterial blood gas (ABG) or via pulse oximetry.

Normal partial pressure of oxygen, as measured via ABG, ranges from about 75-100 millimeters of mercury (mmHg). Values of 60 or less indicate the need for supplemental oxygen.

Oxygen saturation, measured by either ABG or pulse oximetry, is considered normal when it is 95 percent or above. Values of 90 or less indicate the need for supplemental oxygen, although many insurance companies (including Medicare) require a saturation of 88 percent or less to cover supplemental oxygen.

Often, a patient will undergo a six-minute walk test to determine whether they desaturate with activity to qualify them for supplemental oxygen. However, wide variation in testing protocols from facility to facility and clinician to clinician, among other limitations, can lead to imperfect patterns of oxygen prescription and usage.

Shortness of breath does not equal saturation (SaO₂%)

As I say over and over (and over) again, breathing is multifactorial, meaning there are many, many factors besides just the respiratory system and pulmonary function that can affect how well or how poorly we breathe. These include things such as cardiovascular health, level of conditioning (or deconditioning), medications, emotional state, and weather, among others.

Shortness of breath does not always indicate that you are hypoxic. In other words, your level of *dyspnea*, or air hunger, does not always correlate with your oxygen saturation.

This means that you can be short of breath, even extremely short of breath, even in the presence of normal oxygen saturation. Conversely, you can be hypoxic even if you are not particularly short of breath or disproportionately to your shortness of breath. Let's examine what this means to you.

Why am I so short of breath if my oxygen saturation is OK?

One of the most common questions that I am asked is how a person can be so short of breath and yet have a normal oxygen saturation (see above: "Breathing is multi-factorial"). In the case of the individual who is short of breath but has a normal oxygen saturation, *supplemental oxygenation will not help you.* I repeat, if your oxygen saturation is normal, supplemental oxygen will provide little, if any benefit, other than what EMTs and paramedics often refer to as "psychological first aid" or what some medical professionals refer to as "Obecalp" (read it backwards). So, what should you do instead?

In my book, *Ultimate Pulmonary Wellness*, I describe in detail a technique that we call "Recovery from Shortness of Breath." In a nutshell:

1. **Stop what you are doing.** Nobody ever becomes less short of breath by continuing the activity that made them short of breath in the first place. You either must reduce your demand for air or increase your supply. The best way to reduce the demand is to stop whatever it is you're doing.
2. **Talk to yourself, reminding yourself that you know what to do.** Self-talk can be very empowering in high-stakes situations like these (if you do know what to do). If you don't know, I would strongly recommend enrolling in either an in-person or online pulmonary rehabilitation program.
3. **Assume the position.** There are certain positions we call "recovery positions" that will help you to regain control of your breathing. These include several variations of bending over or leaning forward, resting your arms on your thighs or on a stationary object or wall. This allows the abdominal contents to drop forward, improving respiratory mechanics.

4. **Begin controlled breathing techniques (CBT).** These include controlled breathing techniques such as diaphragmatic and pursed-lip breathing, among others. Again, if you are not familiar with these techniques, I would strongly recommend enrolling in a pulmonary rehabilitation program, either in person or online.

5. **Reassess and adapt.** Now that you've caught your breath, reassess the situation and continue the activity (if you can) using the controlled breathing techniques and modifying the activity.

6. In addition to the above, if you have not already done so, now might be a good time to consider using your rescue inhaler (with your doctor's blessing) to further increase your air supply. In an ideal world (and with your doctor's blessing), you might consider pre-medicating approximately 15 minutes before activity.

How can my oxygen be so low if I am not even short of breath?

In the case of the individual who is not particularly short of breath but who is hypoxic as measured either by ABG or pulse oximetry, they *need oxygen*. Again, if your ABG or pulse oximeter indicate you are hypoxic, you need oxygen whether you are short of breath or not. Hypoxia, even in the absence of significant shortness of breath, increases your risk of coronary insufficiency/ischemia, arrhythmia, pulmonary hypertension, and heart failure, among other potential hazards to your health, so as Lung Man says: "Use your oxygen, dammit!"

Rely on your instruments!

Although many people are convinced that they can tell their own oxygen saturation based on how they feel, particularly as it relates to shortness of breath, I liken this to the *"Guesser"* who purports to guess your age, weight, or birth month at the carnival. Keep in mind that in the case of oxygenation, the stakes are much higher than a stuffed animal. And in the same way a SCUBA diver must rely on their depth gauge, or a pilot relies on an altimeter, I always advise people to rely on their instruments, *not the way they feel.*

When (and how often) should I measure my oxygen?

The goal of measuring your oxygen is not to turn you into an obsessive measurement freak. The goal is to make sure you are sufficiently oxygenated both at rest and at *all* levels of activity. This means that at least until you start to understand how your body responds to increasing activity and how much oxygen it takes to keep you saturated, you will have to take more frequent measurements. You might even consider keeping a journal for a while until you can fully assess your body's needs. As you start to understand your body's trends, you can measure less frequently or if you are in distress.

This goes for pulmonary rehabilitation programs as well. I hear from people all the time about rehab programs that measure your oxygen before and after exercise but crickets *during* exercise. Again, if we want to assess a plane's performance *in the air*, we must take our measurements *in the air*, not just before takeoff and after landing.

Myths and misconceptions

Let's also take a few moments to address some of the other myths, misconceptions, misinformation, and miseducation, as well as that famous river in northeast Africa (De Nile).

For the patient that only uses oxygen at home but not when they are out: Many people use their oxygen at home but do not take it with them when they leave the house. This is completely counterintuitive. Again, keeping in mind the principle of supply and demand, the times you need it most is when you are active and most likely to desaturate and contrary to what some people believe, you cannot somehow store oxygen in your body for use later. If — and this is a big IF — you want to "experiment" by not using your oxygen (with your doctor's blessing), the time to do it is when you are at home where the environment is controlled and while you are at rest and the demand is low.

For the patient who "only goes down to 88 percent:" **When** it comes to oxygen saturation, each percentage point is not created equal. Due to the way our hemoglobin takes on and gives up oxygen (as evidenced by the S-shaped oxygen-hemoglobin dissociation curve), as you drop below 90 percent, the magnitude of oxygen change in your bloodstream is greater than when you are between 90 and 100. Think about it like this: You want to take a photo with the Grand Canyon behind you. You are 10 feet from the edge of the canyon. You can go anywhere between 1 and 10 feet with no ill effects, BUT, if you go that 11th foot — you get the idea. It is a similar principle with oxygen saturation. In addition, if we consider the plus or minus 3 percent (or more) error range of most pulse oximeters, a reading of 90 percent can be as low as 87 percent (or less).

For the patient whose oxygen "only goes down for a few minutes" or "recovers quickly:" I told you before that hypoxia increases the risk of many problems including coronary insufficiency/ischemia, arrhythmia, pulmonary hypertension, and heart failure. The risk increases the lower you go, the longer you stay there, and the more frequently you desaturate. But think of it like this. Imagine sitting in a glass booth that suddenly fills up with smoke, but don't worry — it clears very quickly. I think most of us would agree it would be better if it never filled up with smoke in the first place. Well, that is how your brain, heart, and other vital organs feel about hypoxia, so as Lung Man says: "Wear your oxygen, dammit!"

Finally, for the patient who is worried about getting "too much oxygen:" It is for all these previously mentioned reasons that I like my patients to stay at 93 percent or greater during activity. This includes patients with COPD, PF, and PH *including people who are "CO2 retainers."* Every time I say this, people bring up the concept of hypoxic drive and the concern that the patient will stop breathing if we give them too much oxygen.

Basically, the idea behind this theory is that when patients have chronically high levels of carbon dioxide and/or prolonged periods of pH imbalance, they switch over to "hypoxic drive." In other words, instead of responding to high levels of CO_2 or changes in acid-base chemistry, which are the normal stimuli for respiration, they now respond to low oxygen and if we give them "too much oxygen," they will stop breathing all together.

Now again, this is a call that needs to be made by your physician, BUT I can say that in my more than 27 years as both a cardiopulmonary physical therapist and emergency medical technician in many, many different environments, I have never, ever, seen this happen. Neither has Mark. Neither has Ryan. Again, this is *our* experience, but you would think that in a few hundred thousand exercise sessions, one of us would have seen it at least once, especially considering the abundance of supplemental oxygen we use.

In the next section, we will discuss the various devices, accessories and best practices used in the delivery and usage of supplemental oxygen.

Oxygen Manifesto 2: Originally printed in COPD News Today, June 19, 2019

When it comes to home improvement, people typically want three things from a contractor: good, fast, and cheap. Under all but the most rigorous (and lucky) circumstances, you can choose any two of the three. What this means is that you can have it good and fast, but chances are, it's gonna cost you an arm and a leg. And while you may be able to get it fast and cheap, I can assure you that it probably won't be that good. Or you may also be able to get it good and cheap, but it's not gonna be fast. This could be why we can never get in touch with our contractor (once they have your deposit, of course).

There is a similar scenario occurring in the world of supplemental oxygen. People want three things. They want a delivery system that will be small and lightweight. They want a system that will last a long time. And they want a system that will provide a high liter flow, AKA a lot of oxygen.

Well, guess what? You can choose any two. What this means is you can have a system that is lightweight and long- (or more likely, medium-) lasting, but it's not going to give you much oxygen. You can have a system that is lightweight and delivers a lot (or at least a moderate amount) of oxygen, but it's not going to last very long. Or you can have a system that gives you a fair amount of oxygen and lasts for a fair amount of time, but it won't be light.

I tell you these things (as I have for more than three decades) not to scare you nor for the sole purpose of putting the oxygen companies on blast (*although many of them need to be on blast*). I tell you these things because I think it's important for you to understand that the medical oxygen system is rigged, *and not in your favor.* And the systems themselves can be very confusing, even for many clinicians.

It also involves money, and as you know, often when a situation involves money, that's when a lot of wolves; whose primary objective is to line their own pockets; come out in sheep's clothing. Well, think of me as Little Red Riding Hood here to help you see the wolf for who he or she really is and help you get the best oxygen delivery system *for you.*

It's sort of like the Seinfeld episode where Kramer comes up with a coffee table book about coffee tables. Well, it's sad to say, but we need a better supplemental oxygen system for supplemental oxygen systems.

Recently, I received a phone call from a longtime patient named Mrs. M., inquiring about a new portable oxygen concentrator (POC) she was planning to buy *with her own money.* She was told by one of the company's sales agents that the device could provide up to 6 liters per minute (lpm) of oxygen. I assured Mrs. M. that this could not possibly be true because no POC exists that can deliver 6 lpm. She was sure this was what the representative told her, so I asked her to have them call me.

I soon received a phone call from that person's sales manager, who finally and reluctantly conceded that the numbers were manufacturer's settings, not liters per minute. I wondered to myself if this was in fact a light bulb moment for him.

We *eventually* agreed that on a setting of six, the device would provide 1,260 ml of oxygen (1.26 liters) per minute, which I stated would not be enough for Mrs. M.

To be clear, Mrs. M. has been my patient for a very long time, and I have been a cardiopulmonary physical therapist for a very long time (27-plus years). So, when I stated that the POC in question would not meet my patient's needs, I wasn't telling the gentleman what I think. I was telling him what I know.

He then went on to oxygen-splain that that was why there was a 30-day money-back guarantee. *Ohhh.* We also discussed the "re-stocking fee," which he assured me would be waived if the machine did not meet Ms. M.'s needs. *How generous* (yes, while I know you probably find this hard to believe, I am being sarcastic).

Well, guess what? The following week, I tested the device with my patient, and sure enough, it didn't even come close to meeting her needs (as I knew very well it wouldn't).

So now my patient is in the uncomfortable position of having to return the device and, as you can imagine, deeply disillusioned because she was promised a rose garden full of lightweight oxygen that loves you long time.

But there is something even more important that should be considered. We are talking about supplemental oxygen, not a non-stick frying pan, not a mattress, and not a prom dress; oxygen: a crucial life-sustaining substance, without which people can get hurt or die.

Think of it like a parachute or the air bag in your car. If they don't do what they are supposed to do in the way they are supposed to do it, well, that 30-day money-back guarantee really won't be of much use, will it?

It is for all these reasons that my goal is now, as it has always been, to help you gain the greatest understanding of your oxygen requirements, as well as how to ensure that these requirements will be met, so you can truly get the best system *for you* and use it to your maximal advantage. I will explain these concepts using simple terms and descriptions, leaving out the scientific mumbo-jumbo you don't need to know to choose your best device.

The rest of this piece will be composed of concepts that every prospective oxygen user should understand, and you can put them in the bank like money, meaning they are correct. If you don't believe me, you can ask Mark Mangus. If you don't believe Mark, you can ask Ryan Diesem. If you don't believe any of us three, well then just stop reading now because there's really no hope for you. OK. Here we go.

Oxygen by any other name ...

Oxygen can come in one of three basic forms. It can come as a gas, as in a metal tank or cylinder; it can come from a concentrator, which can either be stationary, as in those plug-in home models, or portable (POC); or it can come as a liquid. There are upsides and downsides to each one of these delivery methods, and often, it comes down (or should come down) to making the best choice *for you* (or availability, as is the case of liquid oxygen, which I will discuss at the end).

As a rule, oxygen coming from a tank will be purer than that coming from a stationary concentrator, meaning that 2 (or 3 or 4) lpm from a tank will have a slightly to more than slightly higher percentage of oxygen. In the case of most tanks, this should be 100% medical-grade oxygen and, depending upon the regulator used, can go as high as 25 lpm. When it comes to the home stationary plug-in units, some can go as high as 10 lpm, just slightly less pure than the tanks.

It also means that 3 lpm on a tank will likely keep you slightly (or somewhat more than slightly) more saturated than 3 lpm on a stationary concentrator, and although they are supposed to be equal, I can assure you they are not. Therefore, your oxygen saturation is so much higher on that big, beautiful, green and silver tank you use at rehab compared with your shorter, squatter (think R2-D2), slightly less beautiful concentrator sitting in your living room.

This brings me to my next point, which is why I used 3 lpm as my example. At this moment in time, 3 lpm is the maximum amount of oxygen that can be delivered continuously by *any* POC. *Period.*

While this may not be what you want to hear, it is what you need to hear so that if a sales rep tries to tell you that their unit goes up to 6 lpm, you can say without a doubt that 6 refers to a manufacturer's *setting*, and *not* liters per minute. Any higher number than 3 *refers* to a **manufacturer setting** that *corresponds* to a substantially lower liter flow.

At this moment, liquid oxygen provides the closest we can get to having all three wishes granted by the same unit, in that it's lightweight, has a long duration, and provides high continuous liter flows. In fact, for those reasons, I think a great name for these units would be *The Genie.* The problem is, for most people, genies don't really exist.

Due to a lack of adequate reimbursement from the Center for Medicare and Medicaid Services (CMS) and other third-party payers, liquid oxygen has become increasingly difficult for suppliers to provide and, consequently, nearly impossible for many patients to obtain. I am currently working with a team on a new product and a system that will hopefully solve this problem, but it is also crucial for patient advocacy groups to keep the pressure on Washington.

There are other important factors that would be helpful for you to know about liquid oxygen, but I prefer to address those as an independent subject. Yes, it's that important.

Continuous Versus Pulsed Delivery

As the names imply, continuous oxygen is delivered continuously, meaning it is always flowing. Pulsed-dose oxygen will provide intermittent bursts of oxygen, typically triggered by breathing in through the nose.

All three forms of oxygen (tanks, concentrators, and liquid) can potentially provide both continuous and pulsed oxygen depending upon the device and the accessory equipment used, and if you think about why this is so, it should make perfect sense.

Tanks can run continuously or with the help of a conserving-type regulator. They vary in size and weight and can provide high (or at least moderate) liter flows. These two factors will determine how long they will last. In other words, the larger the tank, the longer it will last. The higher the liter flow, the shorter it will last.

Home (plugin) concentrators can provide high liter flows (up to 10 lpm on some models) due to the increased size and number of sieve beds, the filter that separates the nitrogen from the oxygen in the air. In addition, they don't have the same time constraints as portable units since they run on AC electricity as opposed to a battery. As such, they are neither small, lightweight, nor are they very portable, although most are on wheels so you can move them around the house more easily. Two scenarios you need to be prepared for would be either equipment malfunction or a power outage. So, if you do rely on a home concentrator, please make sure you have a few tanks on hand as a backup.

The single best source I have found related to portable oxygen concentrators, particular the actual devices themselves, is the <u>Pulmonary Paper's</u> annual Portable Oxygen Concentrator Guide, written by respiratory therapist and oxygen super-guru, Ryan Diesem. The guide provides excellent descriptions, as well as specifications, for the vast majority, if not all, available units.

While my goal is never to reinvent the wheel, there are a few points I want to make that will help you use the guide to your maximum advantage in deciding which unit to buy (*or not to buy*) –William Shakespeare.

When comparing POCs with one another and with other delivery systems, be sure to check the *maximum oxygen production* in milliliters (ml) per minute. If you divide this number by 1,000, you will get the maximum amount of oxygen that the unit can produce in liters per minute. As an example, a unit that can produce 3,000 ml per minute produces 3 lpm, regardless of the number of settings it has. A device that produces 1,050 ml per minute provides 1.05 lpm, and a unit that produces 680 ml produces 0.68 lpm, not even 1 lpm. How is that for perspective? For the 2019 guide, Ryan even did the math for you, which is a super-valuable addition.

So, if you require 6 lpm with a non-rebreather mask to stay saturated during your pulmonary rehab sessions, it is highly unlikely that one of these units will meet your needs. In the case of Mrs. M., even though the unit had six settings, the maximum oxygen delivered was still only 1260 ml or 1.26 lpm, which is *one of the reasons* why it couldn't keep her saturated unless she was at rest (which sort of defeats the purpose of a portable unit). We will discuss some of the other reasons in the next installment.

All the above commentary assumes that all other factors are created equal and that they all take place in an ideal world, neither of which is usually the case. For this reason, it is crucial for you to understand the other factors that will either make your device acceptable to you *and* how to get the maximum effectiveness and greatest bang for your buck, regardless of manufacturer, unit, or delivery method.

These include factors such as whether you use a nasal cannula versus a mask, as well as using the correct breathing techniques to ensure the oxygen makes it into your lungs, regardless of the delivery device. These factors will be discussed in the next section, which was the third and final installment of the "Oxygen Manifesto," along with this piece and "Oxygen Manifesto Part 1."

Below is an excerpt from a letter I wrote to an unnamed POC supplier on behalf of my patient. I share this (with Mrs. M.'s permission) to help you to navigate the system more effectively and to help you hold companies more accountable.

To whom it may concern:

Recently, I received a phone call from my longtime patient, Mrs. M. inquiring about your new [insert company and model number here]. She was told by one of your sales agents that the [model] provides up to 6 liters per minute of oxygen. I assured Mrs. M. that this could not possibly be true because there is no POC capable of delivering 6 liters per minute. ...

I then spoke with a manager at your company who began the conversation by stating that the [model] goes up to 6 liters per minute before acquiescing that the numbers were manufacturer's settings and not actually liters per minute. ...

We eventually agreed that the (model) on setting 6 would provide 1,260 ml of oxygen (1.26 liters) per minute, which I stated would not be enough. ... I tested the device with Mrs. M. and sure enough, it didn't even come close to meeting her needs.

So, now, what I would like is for Ms. M. to be able to return this device, no questions asked (because I have answered them all here) and with no restocking fee.

But there is something even more important that I think you should consider. ...

It is crucial from a safety and ethics perspective that your agents first and foremost know and understand the truth; that the pulsed settings on a POC are just that; settings and NOT lpm.

Second, it is crucial from a safety and ethics perspective that your agents share that truth ... with the patient, even if it means acknowledging that the device will likely be insufficient in meeting their needs and therefore, not ship-ping (selling) the device. ...

Also, please keep in mind that when patients are living with a chronic illness, especially one that makes it diffi-cult to breathe, they are willing to try almost anything to reclaim their independence and their lives. This makes them particularly susceptible to high, and sometimes even not-so-high-pressure salesmanship. That's the ethics portion of the equation.

I understand that sometimes (even though they should), patients are not always properly field-tested or educated on exactly how much oxygen they need under which situations or what device will meet those needs. But if a clinician is telling you that it won't, please go ahead and believe them and do the right thing by the patient. ... Please help Mrs. M. smoothly return her [model] without any glitches. ...

Thank you in advance for your cooperation.

YOUR NAME HERE

Oxygen Manifesto 3: Originally printed in Pulmonary Fibrosis News, August 5, 2019

Hell-O$_2$ U, my fellow Oxygen Aficionados! This is the third install-ment of our "Oxygen Manifesto" series.

For this segment, I have enlisted the help of one of my cardiopulmonary physical therapy heroes, mentors, friends, and the mother
of modern-day chest physical therapy and pulmonary rehabilitation, Dr. Donna Frownfelter, and one of my 28-year colleagues,
friends, and chest physical therapy/secretion clearance guru,
Marion Mackles. When I was a physical therapy student in 1992,
we used the second edition of Donna's textbook *Chest Physical
Therapy and Pulmonary Rehabilitation* in our cardiopulmonary
class; we are currently working on the sixth edition.

I hope that through this series, Donna, Marion, Mark Mangus,
Ryan Diesem, and I have succeeded in providing you with valuable
information in a clear, easy-to-understand format you can now use
to help make the best oxygen decisions *for you.*

In these final segments, we want to tie everything together by
discussing some basic concepts that are often overlooked, underes-
timated in their importance, or even unknown, as a way to further
deepen your perspective on supplemental oxygen use, and give you
a few simple "oxygen hacks" and insider tricks of the trade that can
make a huge difference with respect to oxygen use and efficiency
as well as your overall health and wellness. Let's begin.

Pulmonary Anatomy and Physiology

Air can enter the body through either the nose or the mouth. When
you breathe in through your nose, three important functions are
performed. First, the air is filtered by tiny hair-like structures;

called cilia, trapping particles of dust and debris in the mucus membranes. Second and third, the air is warmed and humidified by tiny blood vessels called capillaries.

From the nose, air continues into the nasopharynx, the uppermost part of the throat. When you breathe in through your mouth, air passes through the oropharynx, the middle part of the throat. The nasopharynx and oropharynx meet in the back of the throat, or pharynx, and continue down through the laryngopharynx, the lowest part of your throat and the larynx (also known as the voice box).

From the larynx, air enters the trachea, or windpipe, through the epiglottis, a flap of cartilage that opens during breathing and closes during swallowing to prevent solids and liquids from entering the trachea, airways, and lungs.

The trachea then splits into the right and left mainstem bronchi, going to the right and left lung, respectively. The bronchi then continue to divide, getting smaller and smaller, branching into secondary and tertiary bronchi and even smaller bronchioles. After approximately 20 to 23 divisions, the air finally reaches the alveoli, the tiny air sacs in the lungs where gas exchange occurs.

Efficiency, Effectiveness, and Miles Per Gallon

If you think of your body like a car, the efficiency with which your body uses oxygen is like how many miles you get per gallon of gas (mpg). If you are out of gas, even the most beautiful car will sit idle without fuel to power it. If your engine is run down, your oil badly needs changing, or your tires don't have the proper amount of air in them, your car will be less efficient and get fewer miles per gallon. The same is true when it comes to your body.

Good News!

Here is the good news, though, and again, we are completely biased. But in our experience, we have found that the *right* combination and type of exercise and breathing techniques can significantly improve the effectiveness of the respiratory, cardiovascular, and muscular systems, thereby improving your body's overall efficiency at using oxygen.

In addition, despite a large body of scientific literature stating the opposite, we firmly believe that under the right conditions, your pulmonary function can also improve. In the Exercise chapter of *Ultimate Pulmonary Wellness*, I explain what makes our training methods so different, so effective, and what we believe is the key to improving pulmonary function. Understanding these principles will hopefully allow you, the patient, as well as other rehabilitation professionals and programs, to benefit from what we at the Pulmonary Wellness & Rehabilitation Center *know* to be true.

Ventilation and Respiration

The mechanical act of moving air in and out of the lungs, i.e., inhalation and exhalation, is called ventilation. Ventilation is an *active* process, meaning it requires the contraction and relaxation of the respiratory muscles for it to occur.

The chemical exchange of oxygen (O_2) and carbon dioxide (CO_2) between the external environment and the cells of the body is called respiration or gas exchange. Respiration is a passive process and occurs constantly, regardless of muscle activity or phase of ventilation. In other words, it occurs at the cellular level, during both inhalation and exhalation, as well as during any pauses in between.

Breathing Pattern is Still King (or Queen)

Regardless of whether you use supplemental oxygen or not, breathing pattern will play the greatest role in how well or how poorly we breathe. When we are talking about breathing pattern, we are referring to variables such as your respiratory rate, rhythm, and depth, as well as which muscles are being used. Our breathing pattern can be affected by many factors including our anatomy (i.e., "normal chest wall" versus a scoliosis, or pectus excavatum, or asymmetry, which can occur in a person who has had a stroke), physiology and pathophysiology, pain, environment, and even our emotions, among many others.

Respiratory Rhythm

Normal, unlabored breathing (also sometimes called quiet breathing) is known as eupnea and should be regular or steady. Abnormal, irregular, or labored breathing is called dyspnea, and is closely related to a person's shortness of breath (SOB) or perception of breathlessness.

Musculature and Symmetry

During normal breathing, the chest and abdomen should rise and fall together as the diaphragm, the main inspiratory muscle, contracts, and the lungs fill up with air. The initial movement is seen in the upper abdomen just below the xiphoid process, the lateral lower chest moves up and out to the sides, and if the breath is large, the upper chest will move. In quiet breathing, basically the upper abdomen and rib cage move. It is when we take deeper breaths, we see the upper chest move. The same is true for when the diaphragm relaxes, and the lungs expel air.

During labored breathing, accessory muscles of the neck, shoulders, chest, and back can be recruited. Other signs of distress might include nasal flaring or tripod position, in which a person will lean forward with his or her elbows on the thighs when in a seated position, or bending over, leaning forward on the upper extremities (or something else) when standing.

Generally, both sides (right and left) of the chest should move symmetrically or equally. An asymmetrical breathing pattern is abnormal and can indicate a physical or physiological problem.

Respiratory Rate (RR)

Respiratory rate (RR) refers to how many breaths we take per minute, i.e., how fast (or slow) we breathe. In adults, normal respiratory rate is 12 or in some references, 10–20 breaths per minute. A respiratory rate of greater than 20 breaths per minute is called tachypnea and a respiratory rate of less than 12 breaths per minute is called bradypnea.

Depth or Tidal Volume (TV or V_t)

Depth of breathing refers to how shallow or deep we are breathing and represents the inspiratory, or tidal volume (TV or Vt), i.e., the amount of air we breathe in and out with each breath.

Minute Volume (MV)

Minute ventilation can be described as the amount of air we breathe in and out in one minute and can be represented as RR x TV, in other words, the number of breaths we take per minute multiplied by the amount of air we breathe in and out with each breath.

Overcoming the Trachea

The trachea, or windpipe, is known as anatomical dead space because, as opposed to being able to perform gas exchange, it is simply a conduit and does not allow oxygen to enter the blood where it can be used by the body. Think of it like a jet bridge, the corridor at the airport that takes you from the waiting area at the gate to the plane. You can be anywhere along that 150-foot tunnel, but unless you make it onto the plane, you're not going anywhere. It is, in fact, just a conduit that must be passed for our breathing to be effective.

The volume of air in the trachea can very roughly be thought of as approximately as many milliliters as your weight in pounds, so for the purposes of this example, we will use a 150-pound person, and therefore, the trachea will account for 150 milliliters of air.

6 Liters Per Minute

On average, most of us breathe approximately 6–8 liters per minute (6,000–8,000 milliliters). If we use that as our standard to think about the impact of respiratory rate, you will see the following:

If you breathe at a respiratory rate of 12 breaths per minute (low end of normal), each breath would be 500 milliliters. With that in mind, for every 500-milliliter breath, 150 milliliters are used to bypass the trachea and 350 milliliters per breath, or 4,200 milliliters per minute, make it into the lungs where it can be used by the body.

$$6{,}000 \div 12 = 500 - 150 = 350$$

If you breathe at a respiratory rate of 20 breaths per minute (high end of normal), each breath would be 300 milliliters. With that in mind, for every 300-milliliter breath, 150 milliliters are used to bypass the trachea and 150 milliliters per breath, or 3,000 milliliters per minute, make it into the lungs where it can be used by the body.

$$6{,}000 \div 20 = 300 - 150 = 150$$

If you breathe at a respiratory rate of 40 breaths per minute (high), each breath would be 150 milliliters. With that in mind, for every 150-milliliter breath, 150 milliliters are used to bypass the trachea, and none of that makes it into the lungs where it can be used by the body.

$$6000 \div 40 = 150 - 150 = 0$$

Is it any wonder you feel so bad or that your oxygen plummets when you are panting like a dog trying to catch your breath? This highlights the importance of trying to take slow deep breaths using controlled breathing techniques, as described in *Ultimate Pulmonary Wellness*, such as pursed-lip breathing, diaphragmatic breathing, paced breathing, and recovery from shortness of breath methods for those "code red" situations.

This is always true, but even more so if you require supplemental oxygen because as you can see from the above, regardless of what device you use or what setting or liter flow you have it on, if you are breathing at 40 breaths per minute, it's not going to do you much good because the oxygen won't get into the lungs where you can use it. And this is especially, especially true in the case of a pulsed-delivery system. Don't stop the breath as soon as you hear the device trigger. Breathe deeply so that the oxygen makes it into the lungs where your body can use it.

As an adjunct to the above techniques, try this "Donna Frownfelter Special," which should help you to decrease your respiratory rate and give you greater control of your breathing. Take a short pause (one to two seconds) at the top of inspiration and at the end of exhalation. To be clear, this should not be a breath-holding maneuver, just a slight inspiratory and expiratory pause.

And here is an additional pearl from chest physical therapist extraordinaire, Marion Mackles. During exhalation, instead of just trying to blow the air out or allowing the air to escape gently through pursed lips, place your hands on your knees with your elbows out (bulldog position), and allow your body to slowly collapse forward as you sigh out through pursed lips. As you start to inhale again, push up gently on your arms as you return your upper body to the upright position. By folding the thorax over the abdomen like an accordion, the increased pressure from the abdominal contents assists in expelling the air from your lungs and helps in setting up your next inhalation.

Chapter 9:

Ultimate Pulmonary Wellness by Noah Greenspan, PT, DPT, CCS, EMT-B

"The whole is greater than the sum of its parts." – **Aristotle**

In today's healthcare environment, an overwhelming percentage of resources are spent on treating diseases and their associated manifestations. While treatment of disease is an essential part of wellness, there is far more to being healthy than simply not being sick. Instead of merely trying to eliminate illness, true *wellness* is the goal we are striving for—and can be achieved through a combination of positive life changes, education, and enlightenment, all of which can have a potentially powerful impact on both disease treatment and *prevention*.

With that in mind, my goal is always to present you with the information that I have found to be the *most* successful and *most* practical over the past 30 years as well as to help guide you in determining which ones will work and which ones won't work *for you*.

If you read the classic literature on pulmonary rehabilitation, you will find hundreds of articles stating that after participation in a pulmonary rehabilitation program, participants feel better, can do more, and are less short of breath. However, most of these same articles will also state that pulmonary rehabilitation *does not* improve pulmonary function, which can often be disappointing for people.

Even though we do not necessarily agree with these findings, what this tells us is that if you feel better, can do more, and are less short of breath, without any improvement in pulmonary function, there must be other factors involved in how well or how poorly you breathe—things like fitness level, nutrition, and emotional state. This is great news because these are things that we have some control over.

In this chapter, we will set the stage for the next several months, years, and hopefully the rest of your life, by identifying the *most* important principles of Ultimate Pulmonary Wellness.

Let's start with a few definitions:

Ultimate: The dictionary defines "ultimate" as consummate, maximum, most, or to the highest degree or quantity. Sounds impressive, right? I would also add "quality" to this description because I hear people say repeatedly—and I also believe—that *quality* of life is equally if not more important than quantity. Our goal is not just for you to feel pretty good. Our goal is for you to feel *amazing* and to achieve the absolute maximal level of health, function, and quality of life possible.

Pulmonary: "Pulmonary" pertains to the lungs and the respiratory system. When I ask people to rate their understanding of their condition or even the basics of the respiratory system, most people report around a C+ grade level. I don't know about you but if you're living with a chronic pulmonary disease and you have only a C+ understanding of the respiratory system, I consider this a problem.

In an ideal world, when you receive a diagnosis like Pulmonary Fibrosis, IPF, ILD, or any other medical condition, it would be great if you could spend an hour or two with your doctor, asking questions and taking notes about all the things that you need to know.

However, in today's fast-paced healthcare environment, doctors are often so busy that even the greatest, most caring physicians simply do not have the time to teach you everything that you need to know about your illness. That's our other motivation for writing this book.

Wellness: Often, when we seek medical care, we are focused on the exact opposite of wellness. In fact, as a society, we spend far more resources battling sickness than promoting true wellness. Typically, when patients first report their symptoms to their doctor (shortness of breath, cough, or the inability to walk uphill), the first treatments will almost always be medication (or more likely, medications).

However, not enough thought is given to the other factors that come into play when it comes to breathing. Lifestyle choices can either make you feel better or worse depending on which ones you choose to do—or not do—things like exercise, eating a healthier diet, quitting smoking, taking steps to manage stress and anxiety, and *prevention* of infection.

The Formula

Ultimate Pulmonary Wellness (UPW) can be divided into five major categories, with each one accounting for *approximately* 20% of total pulmonary and overall health. Those 5 categories are Medical, Exercise, Nutrition, Management of Stress and Anxiety, and Prevention of Infection.

I will touch on these areas briefly in this chapter to give you an overview of the program and to highlight the role of each of these components in your health and well-being. Later in the book, there will be a chapter for each topic that goes into much greater detail and gives you specific guidelines and suggestions for each.

Medical (20%)

To me, good medicine means having the right doctor or doctors, taking the right medications, and taking those medications properly. People ask me all the time "How do you know if you have the right doctor?" At the most basic level, you probably want a doctor who is smart, experienced, and compassionate. After that, most of us look for any variety of other qualities and character traits. What characteristics do you look for in a doctor? We will help you clarify some of your own physician "makes" or "breaks."

When it comes to medications, taking the proper medicines is heavily dependent upon having the right doctor but getting the most benefit from your medicines also depends upon taking them properly, as well as using the delivery devices properly. We will discuss these topics in greater detail later in the book.

Exercise (20%)

When we discussed shortness of breath, we talked about the fact that people often avoid activities that cause them shortness of breath. Consequently, all the muscles that you use to do those activities get weaker and your body becomes less efficient at using oxygen. In addition to teaching you specific breathing exercises, I will guide you through the most beneficial exercises and help you put together a program that will be most effective and best suited *for you*.

Nutrition (20%)

When it comes to nutrition, in addition to eating a balanced and healthy diet, there are certain concepts that relate particularly to pulmonary disease. These include topics like mechanics of eating and breathing or being at your correct (healthy) weight. In addition, there are certain foods that will help you fight your disease and its associated symptoms, while others will make them worse.

Stress, Anxiety, and Depression Management (20%)

Stress, anxiety, and depression can have a devastating impact on someone living with a pulmonary disease. To make matters worse, living with a pulmonary disease can cause a tremendous amount of anxiety and depression. This is another cycle that we hope to break so that you can be less stressed and live a happier, healthier, more satisfying life.

Prevention of Infection (20%)

The final piece of the puzzle is prevention of infection. To be clear, a cold, flu, or other infection for someone with a respiratory disease can be far more serious than for someone who is otherwise healthy. Plus, people with lung disease often don't get a little infection. They get big infections, and their infections often go right to the chest.

Because the respiratory system is your weak link, it is crucial that you implement some type of *prevention* strategy. This effort will be well worth your while, as it is often easier to prevent an infection than to treat one once you've got it. I will give you several tools and suggestions to help you in your fight against infection.

One very interesting and very positive bit of news is that thankfully, during the Covid-19 pandemic, I have known of very few patients in our cardiopulmonary patient and caregiver community that contracted Covid. I would like to think that I had at least a tiny role in that, having been training our troops for years on how to prevent infections and the good news is that all the same things that help prevent colds, flus, and other infections, also prevent Covid.

Everything Else (10–100%)

Since we always believe in giving 110% effort, there is an additional 10% left over for a category I like to call "everything else." What I mean by "everything else" is that even if you do everything right including these "*big five*" items of pulmonary wellness, there will always be factors outside of our control. Being superstitious by nature, I don't want to name any of them here but take a deep breath, keep living your life, and expect the unexpected.

How to Use This Formula

Now, let's take each of these "big five" one at a time and expand upon them in a way that will give you a very clear and comprehensive understanding of what factors will help you live a better life and which ones might make your life more difficult. This book is organized so you can go chapter by chapter or you can choose to skip around. So, please, make yourself comfortable and feel free to use the information in whatever fashion makes the most sense to you.

Chapter 10:

Medications by Noah Greenspan, PT, DPT, CCS, EMT-B and Robert J. Kaner, MD

"Drugs don't work if patients don't take them (properly)." – *Former US Surgeon General, C. Everett Koop, MD*

The medical treatment for ILD's can be as diverse and complex as the conditions themselves. This is yet another reason why it behooves you to seek out a physician who truly specializes in the science *and art* of caring for patients with ILD's and a COE.

One crucial point is that for most ILD's there are no cures and, in some cases, few if any treatments will have a direct impact on the progression of the disease or the lungs themselves. In conditions in which the inflammatory trigger is known, it is imperative that the offending agent be removed completely and if it cannot, may require removing yourself from the environment. In still other causes of ILD, the treatment is targeted toward the underlying cause or condition, thereby hoping to improve the respiratory component of the disease and its associated symptoms.

In all these cases, outcome and prognosis with respect to disease severity and life expectancy is highly dependent upon early and correct diagnosis, and specific targeted treatment. For that reason, what you can, could, or should do is way beyond the scope of this book and its authors. Rather, we will give a basic and brief description of some of the medications available to treat ILD's with the super caveat that every treatment regimen must be expertly tailored to the individual patient, based upon their individual condition, and monitored and modified by their own ILD specialists.

NOTE: As you read this chapter, please keep in mind that like any medication, there are often many potential side effects. Therefore, any decisions about potential risks and benefits must be decided with your own physician(s).

Corticosteroids (Prednisone)

Corticosteroids, also known simply as "steroids" are *anti-inflammatories* that can reduce symptoms by suppressing the activity of the immune system, decreasing inflammation and edema (swelling) in the airways, lungs, and other body parts.

Mycophenolate mofetil/mycophenolic acid (Brand Names: Cellcept and Myfortic)

Mycophenolate is an *immunosuppressant* that has anti-inflammatory and anti-fibrotic properties. It can reduce symptoms by suppressing the activity of the immune system. In some cases, this medication can help reduce the need for corticosteroids.

Azathioprine (Brand Name: Imuran)

Azathioprine is an immunosuppressant that reduces symptoms by suppressing the activity of the immune system to prevent the body's immune system from attacking its own cells, that can lead to pulmonary fibrosis. It is often used to treat pulmonary fibrosis and other conditions that cause pulmonary fibrosis, like Rheumatoid Arthritis. In some cases, this medication can help reduce the need for corticosteroids and is often used when other medications are poorly tolerated due to side effects.

Cyclophosphamide (Brand Name: Cytoxan)

Cyclophosphamide is a chemotherapeutic/anti-inflammatory agent that can reduce symptoms by suppressing the activity of the immune system to prevent the body's immune system from attacking its own cells, by destroying specific inflammatory cells in the body. In some cases, this medication can help reduce the need for corticosteroids, or can be used in combination with corti-costeroids or in cases when corticosteroids are contraindicated.

Pirfenidone (Brand Names: Esbriet, Pirfenex, Pirespa)

Although the exact mechanism of action of Pirfenidone is not completely understood, it seems to have anti-inflammatory and anti-fibrotic effects. Pirfenidone does not reverse fibrosis. However, it *may* slow the progression of fibrosis in *some* patients

with PF/IPF. This is another argument for early diagnosis and treatment.

Nintedanib (Brand Name: Ofev)

Nintedanib has anti-inflammatory and anti-fibrotic effects. It acts on the pathways that cause scarring in the lungs in *some* patients with PF/IPF, and scleroderma associated ILD. Nintedanib does not reverse fibrosis. However, it *may* slow the progression of fibrosis in *some* patients with mild to moderate PF/IPF.

Tocilizumab (Brand Name: Actemra)

Tocilizumab is a biologic medication that has anti-inflammatory effects. It *may* slow the rate of decline of pulmonary function in *some* patients with PF/IPF, and scleroderma associated ILD.

Once again, the medical treatment for ILD's can be as diverse and complex as the conditions themselves. This is yet another reason why it behooves you to seek out a physician who truly specializes in the science *and art* of caring for patients with ILD's and a COE.

Rituximab (Brand Name: Rituxan)

Rituximab may offer a safe and effective therapeutic intervention in a subgroup of patients with severe, progressive ILD unresponsive to conventional immunosuppressive medications. It is the go-to for people failing standard therapy for scleroderma, myositis, and other Connective Tissue Disorders (CTD's).

Chapter 11:

Exercise by Noah Greenspan, PT, DPT, CCS, EMT-B

"A body at rest will remain at rest and a body in motion will remain in motion, unless acted upon by an external force." – Sir Isaac Newton's First Law of Motion

One of my absolute core beliefs is that when it comes to health and wellness, exercise is by far, one of, if not *the* single best, most effective lifestyle change you can make and one of the most powerful tools to improve your health as well as your overall quality of life. By going from sedentary to active or from active to more active, you can *reasonably* expect to see improvements in many of your individual physical and physiological systems, as well as your body, and dare I say, your mind and spirit as well. I realize that this may seem a bit cliché (which I usually hate) or new age (which I don't hate at all), but in this case, it happens to be true.

A basic fact of *most* exercise programs for *most* people is that you will generally get out of it what you put into it. Another basic fact is that not all people are created equal. Therefore, not all programs will have the same impact on everyone.

For all these reasons, I would be doing you a tremendous disservice if I were to tell you "This is exactly what *you* should be doing". Instead, I will teach the *principles* that have been most successful for the greatest number of patients at the Pulmonary Wellness & Rehabilitation Center. I'll also show you how to evaluate and make adaptations to your own program to ensure maximum safety, effectiveness and hopefully, maybe even a little fun.

PROFESSIONAL AND LEGAL DISCLAIMER: As I mention time and time again, my patients' safety is my first, second and third priority. Therefore, as with any lifestyle change, please *do not* begin *any* exercise program under the misguided pretense that "Noah told me to do this" or "Noah told me to do that." I did not, I am not, and I will not tell you what *you* should do. So please, regardless of *anything* you read in this book, *always* discuss *any* lifestyle changes you plan to make with your physician before you begin.

Why Exercise?

Exercise can increase not only the pumping power of your heart and the efficiency with which your body utilizes oxygen (which pretty much, everyone knows) but also, the mechanics of your respiratory system and lung function (which, not everyone believes). Exercise also strengthens your skeletal muscles, increases your bone density, reduces body fat, regulates blood sugar and blood pressure, elevates your mood, etcetera, etcetera, etcetera. And it makes you feel good! Maybe not at the exact moment you're doing it, but when done right, the benefits of exercise will far outweigh any minor discomfort you may experience in carrying out your actual workout.

Notice that I said *done right*, because like anything else; if you do it wrong—and there are *plenty* of people doing it wrong—not only will you not achieve the best results, but you could do yourself harm.

"The First Cut is the Deepest"

I often say that the first minute in the gym is the hardest—in other words, just getting there. So, go. When I used to work at NYU, I had a daily dilemma. Every afternoon, when I arrived at the corner of 34th Street and Third Avenue, I could either continue 1 more block up 34th Street and go to the gym, or I could turn right on Third Avenue and go home to watch TV, eat, and sleep. It was quite literally a daily struggle. So, trust me. *I understand*. After all, if exercising were fun and easy, everyone would be in great shape.

However, for most people, once they're at the gym (or physical therapy, or cardiopulmonary rehab), they usually don't seem to mind it so much and they almost always feel better afterward. So, like Nike says, "Just do it." I would take that axiom a step further and say, "Just do something"—*anything*, almost because it *almost* doesn't matter which type of exercise you choose (within reason) if you do some form of activity every day. In other words, show up. So, get up out of your chair or off the couch and haul your butt over to the gym, park, mall, rehabilitation center, your basement or living room, or wherever else it is that inspires you to move your body.

AND...if you don't have access to any of these facilities (and even if you do), we have created our own Pulmonary Wellness Bootcamp which is a FREE 42-day online cardiopulmonary

rehabilitation program that can be done from anywhere...and it's awesome! Bootcamp consists of Thoughts, Motivations, Cardio, Breathing, Balance, Flexibility and Strength training along with Yoga, Tai Chi, Qigong. Meditation, and a whole host of other activities with top experts in the field of cardiopulmonary rehabilitation.

Here's the link: https://pulmonarywellness.org/bootcamp /

A basic rule of physical fitness (and physics) is that your body gets good at doing what you ask it to do. So, if you ask yourself to sit on the couch, eating donuts and flipping the remote (ooh, that sounds nice), that's what your body will get good at. If this is the *"work-out"* you choose, you will find yourself *"rewarded"* with increased stores of adipose tissue (fat); decreased muscle size, strength, and efficiency; increased shortness of breath; and a decrease in your overall aerobic capacity along with thinning bones and a whole host of *negative* adaptations to inactivity. A sedentary lifestyle is also a well-known *modifiable* risk factor for atherosclerosis and coronary artery disease (CAD).

Conversely, if you ask your body to get moving—whether you choose to walk, run, cycle, swim, participate in a formal pulmonary rehab program or any one of the many other potential exercise options—your body will get good at doing those activities, and you will soon find yourself *really* rewarded with *decreased* fat stores, *increased* muscle size, strength and efficiency; *decreased* shortness of breath; and an *increase* in your overall aerobic capacity, along with *increased* bone density and a whole host of *positive* adaptations to activity. In addition, an active lifestyle *reduces* your risk for atherosclerosis and coronary disease. I vote for what's behind door number two.

In this chapter, I will explain how to implement these practices safely and effectively, and as hip-hop legend, Biggie Smalls once said, "go from negative to positive, and it's all good." With that in mind, my goals for this chapter include:

1. To help you understand how to assess your current (baseline) fitness level.
2. To help you start an exercise program that will be the safest and most effective program *for you.*
3. To help you stay motivated and on course with your program.

Let's go!

Exercise Versus Activity

When I ask people whether they exercise, they often tell me that while they don't participate in any type of "formal" exercise program, they are "*very active.*" When I inquire further, they usually tell me they do a lot of cleaning or grocery shopping (or some other activity of daily living).

Don't get me wrong. It's great that you're doing these things. However, most people require more than this type of basic everyday activity to achieve the maximum benefit from exercise. Therefore, for the purposes of this chapter, while we will include these daily tasks in your overall activity count, we will not consider them "exercise."

In most cases, your program should almost always include a more formal (or at least somewhat *structured*) exercise regime in which you exercise solely for the sake of exercise, regardless of your starting point. In addition, for your exercise program to be the most effective (or even effective at all) certain parameters must be followed.

I often ask people to think of their health as a savings account. Using this analogy, every time you do something good for yourself, it's like putting money in the bank. In this case, we are talking about exercise or activity, but this can also include things like meditating, getting a massage, eating a healthy meal, *throwing away those cigarettes*, or any number of things you can do to take better care of yourself.

Conversely, every time you do something that is not so healthy (or downright unhealthy), like spending the whole day in front of the TV, eating a box of cookies, or smoking a cigarette, think of that as making a withdrawal and in some extreme cases, *hemorrhaging* money.

In the same way that your financial goal is to accumulate as much wealth as possible, the same should be true with respect paid to your "health wealth." It is also important to realize that some deposits will be greater than others, meaning that some activities will be more valuable and produce greater benefits than others.

As an example, going for a 20-minute walk will be more valuable than washing the dishes. Every little bit helps, and I would never want to discourage you from participating in any activity that you want (or need) to do (like washing the dishes).

Another thing to realize is that not every day is created equal. Some days will be better than others. This can be dependent upon many, many factors, like the weather, whether you've had a good night's sleep, what or how much you've eaten (or not eaten), and a whole host of other potential factors, some of which will vary significantly from individual to individual and some that will be more universal. This is true regardless of whether you have a pulmonary condition or not.

So, if you happen to be having a particularly bad day, maybe you will only be able to deposit a dollar or a quarter or even a penny. This is still better than nothing. Except in rare instances, doing something, no matter how small, will *always* be better than doing nothing. In fact, as one of my yoga instructors used to say: "as long as you're giving 100% effort, you're still getting 100% of the benefit." Thanks, Stephanie! On the flip side, on the days that you feel great, you can take advantage of it by increasing your activity. On these days, since you're feeling particularly flush, perhaps you can deposit a fiver, a ten or even a twenty-dollar bill.

Activity, Inactivity, and Shortness of Breath

As you know by now, the efficiency with which your body utilizes oxygen depends on three main systems: the respiratory system, or the ability of your lungs to move air in and out; the cardiovascular system, or the ability of your heart to pump blood; and the muscular or musculoskeletal system, the ability of your skeletal muscles to extract and utilize oxygen from the blood. The more active you are, the more efficient each of these systems will become (and vice versa). The less active you are, the less efficient each of these systems will become.

Considering these facts, patients often describe the *dyspnea cycle* as a "downward spiral," or they tell me that they are "going downhill". The good news is that in the same way that you can "spiral downhill," your body's abilities can actually improve with activity, and in many, if not most cases, you can actually start to *"spiral uphill"* again.

Please keep in mind that there are thousands of opinions out there based on people's personal and professional experiences with exercise, as well as a multitude of other factors that go into promoting one form, philosophy, or product versus another. In fact, it can be dizzying listening to the "experts" argue over which is "the best" form of exercise and how it should be done. I will provide you with what I believe is the most beneficial information based upon 30 years of experience working with pulmonary patients. It's up to you to take it from there.

To help you gain a clear understanding of the factors involved in maximizing your exercise program, I have divided this exercise chapter into three parts. The first section will discuss general principles of exercise, like frequency, intensity, type, and time of exercise (FITT). This will provide you with a general overview of which variables are important in establishing the most effective program for you and how each one can be adjusted to give you the most effective workout.

The second part will address what we call exercise testing and prescription. In this portion, I'll explain the basic principles of establishing a baseline and creating the most effective program for you.

Finally, I will walk you through the process I follow when I see a new patient and show you how we create individualized exercise programs based on the data obtained during our initial meeting. Oh, and... Pulmonary Wellness Bootcamp!

The FITT Principle of Exercise

When people discuss exercise programs, we often hear about the *FITT principle*, which stands for *Frequency* of exercise, *Intensity* of exercise, *Type* of exercise and *Time* or duration of exercise. In other words, how often should I exercise, how hard should I exercise, what exercises should I do and how long should I do them for? Basically, these are the four modifiable variables that can be adjusted depending upon your current fitness level and your desired outcome. First, I will discuss each of these variables individually and then I will put them together into sample workouts for you as they specifically relate to people living with lung disease, so that you can begin to develop your own personal exercise program.

Part of the problem is that exercise recommendations are often too general in nature. Also, let's be honest. I can tell you whatever I want to tell you and regardless of what I recommend, you can still choose to do (or not do) whatever you want. For example, I can say "use the exercise bike three times per week for 45 minutes" but if you hate the exercise bike, then you're probably not going to do it. Trust me when I say that I have seen (and owned) many very expensive clothes hangers in my time. For that reason, I've instead chosen to describe several different options for you as well as to explain what you can reasonably expect from each, and then, allow you to decide what works best *for you*.

FREQUENCY OF EXERCISE

When the question of how often people should exercise comes up, you will often hear a wide range of recommendations from the once a week "miracle" to what seems like eight days a week. For general health and fitness benefits, you will most often hear people say three to five days per week (which is *approximately* what I will say). If we are talking about Pulmonary Wellness Bootcamp, the goal is 42 days straight.

In my experience, people feel best and make the most progress when they do *some form* of exercise every day or *almost* every day. This doesn't mean that every day must be spent in the gym or at pulmonary rehab. In fact, it shouldn't. I often tell people that "you do rehab you so you can live your life"—not the other way around.

Here is an exercise myth buster: Many people believe that the body requires a full day of rest between workouts. This is not actually the case. In fact, daily exercise is even more important for people who are sicker or more physically deconditioned. This may seem counterintuitive. However, there are several strong arguments in favor of daily exercise:

1. Depending upon how weak or deconditioned you are; you may only be able to tolerate very short periods of low-intensity exercise. Since these initial workouts will be shorter and less intense, your body will require less recovery time in between workouts.
2. Because these workouts will be shorter and less intense you will need to do them more frequently to gain some momentum. Remember that a body at rest will remain at rest. Also, if you think back to your savings account, because you are making smaller deposits, you will need to make more of them if you want to see your savings grow. Therefore, you may need to do your exercise every day or in some cases, more than once per day. For example, a patient in the hospital might need to go for a walk two to three times per day or every couple of hours to build up their strength and endurance. Likewise, a homebound

patient may need to do their chair exercises two to three times per day or walk around their living room once an hour.

3. As I mentioned previously, your body gets good at doing what you ask it to do. Therefore, you must ask your body to become more active by exercising more frequently. This will offset the amount of time spent lying in bed and counteract the detrimental effects of inactivity. Think about trying to get a stalled car moving. Initially, it takes a much greater push to get it moving, and then momentum kicks in. It's similar with exercise.

At PWRC, our patients participate in formal cardiopulmonary exercise sessions two, three, or four days per week, depending upon their condition. As previously mentioned, Bootcamp is a 42-day program in which you will be exercising daily. As you get stronger and your workouts become longer and more intense, you may need more recovery time or to vary the types of workouts to prevent injury, ensure your safety and make sure you are getting the maximum benefit out of your program. As I mentioned, people do best when they do *some form* of exercise every day or *almost* every day, but I am also a realist and I know that sometimes life can get in the way.

NOTE: It is *crucial* that you listen to your doctor, your health care team, and *your body*. And unless you are doing Bootcamp, always start with the minimum effective dose of exercise—in this case, two days per week—before gradually increasing to greatly minimize the chance of any musculoskeletal injury, cardiovascular event, or any other adverse effect that could potentially be associated with exercise.

INTENSITY OF EXERCISE

When it comes to the intensity of exercise, we are referring to how hard you are working or the percentage of your maximum (actual or predicted) workload. There are many ways to measure the intensity of your workout including both objective and subjective criteria. *Objective* criteria include those that can be observed, counted, measured, or otherwise quantified by an instrument or outside source such as heart rate, blood pressure, or oxygen saturation. However, the objective data is only half the story.

Subjective criteria include things like your personal perception of what you are feeling and experiencing internally. The subjective data—what you're feeling with respect to breathlessness, rating of perceived exertion, as well as any other symptoms or sensations you may be experiencing—is equally, *if not more* important in gaining a complete understanding of your condition. By taking all these factors into consideration, we can maximize your safety and ensure the greatest effectiveness within each workout.

Objective Measures of Exercise Intensity

Maximum Heart Rate:

One of the most common ways that we can represent the intensity of exercise or activity is by the percentage of your maximum heart rate (HR Max%). This method is often very effective, but it can also be equally ineffective depending upon how the numbers are derived. Let me explain why I say this.

Your maximum heart rate is the maximum number of times your heart can beat per minute when you are working at your highest level of exertion or activity. It is based primarily on your age and level of conditioning. Generally, as we age, our maximum heart rate decreases and as another general rule, the more conditioned we are, the lower your heart rate will be, both at rest and at any given workload.

The Theoretical, The Actual and the "Actual" Actual

Your *theoretical* age-predicted maximum heart rate is most often calculated using the formula 220 minus your age (220-age). For example, a 60-year-old person has a *theoretical* age-predicted maximum heart rate of 160 beats per minute (bpm).

However, it is important to understand that this age-predicted formula for maximum heart rate is a theoretical *approximation* based upon *general* population data. It is not an individually established calculation based on your or any one person's distinct set of medical, physical, or other physiological characteristics.

Furthermore, this approximation should only be used as a predictor in "normal, healthy individuals." It does not apply to and therefore, should not be used for "high risk" populations, including anyone with any type of cardiovascular, pulmonary, metabolic, or otherwise significant medical condition that might impair normal exercise physiology or compromise safety.

In clinical or medical settings, we cannot and should not be using the theoretical maximum heart rate. Instead, we need to establish an *actual* maximum heart rate for each individual patient. For that reason, it is strongly recommended that the patient undergo a comprehensive cardiovascular workup prior to beginning an exercise or rehabilitation program, especially in these special cardiopulmonary populations.

At a *minimum*, depending on the number and degree of risk factors, some type of clinical exercise evaluation or stress test (preferably, with an echocardiogram) should be performed to determine the patient's *actual* maximum heart rate as well as to establish safe parameters for exercise. However, here is where things get interesting (and tricky and confusing). When it comes to pulmonary patients, even the actual maximum heart rate does not always apply either.

During a traditional stress test, the exercise would typically be terminated when the patient reaches what we call a *hemodynamic* or *physiologic endpoint*. Usually, these endpoints are based on the patient's age, gender, fitness level, and medical condition, particularly the presence of any potential cardiac risk factors. These endpoints most frequently include heart rate (HR) or pulse in beats per minute (bpm), heart rhythm via electrocardiogram (ECG or EKG), blood pressure (BP) in millimeters of mercury (mm Hg), aerobic capacity or peak oxygen consumption (VO2 max) and in the case of pulmonary patients, oxygen saturation (O2 Sat%).

The test is usually stopped once any one of these pre-determined endpoints is reached, or for any number of other reasons including chest pain, tachycardia (high heart rate), hyper- or hypotension (high or low blood pressure respectively), equipment malfunction, or at the patient's request.

However, it is important to understand that patients with pulmonary disease are often prevented from reaching their true maximum because they are limited by shortness of breath and/or lower extremity fatigue, long before they reach any of these physiologic endpoints. For example, that 60-year-old man might have to stop the test because he is too short of breath to continue even though his heart rate is only 120 as opposed to his age-predicted maximum heart rate of 160. In this scenario, instead of an *actual* maximum heart rate, we get what we call a *symptom-limited* maximum heart rate.

In traditional cardiac rehabilitation programs, an exercise prescription might include a target heart rate (THR) somewhere between 50% and 90% of maximum, depending on the individual's medical history, their current level of conditioning and their personal health and fitness goals. However, this is not usually effective in a pulmonary population or in any patient who is limited by their symptoms prior to being limited by their cardiovascular condition or hemodynamic performance. Another point to make is that many of the medications used to treat pulmonary patients can have a stimulant effect. As a result, in addition to the increased work of breathing and deconditioning, pulmonary patients can sometimes have elevated heart rates, both at rest as well as during exercise.

Metabolic Equivalents (METs)

A Measure of Exercise Tolerance or Metabolic Equivalent (MET) is a unit of measure used to describe cardiovascular workload. One MET equals 3.5 ml $O2 \cdot kg^{-1} \cdot min^{-1}$. In English, this means that for each metabolic equivalent or MET, your body utilizes 3.5 milliliters of oxygen per kilogram of body weight per minute. To take this one step further, each person's body uses a certain amount of oxygen per minute, depending upon the activity they are doing, their body weight and composition, and their fitness level.

We can determine the exact MET level at which a person is working either by direct measurement (using what we call expired gas analysis) or by using predicted values. During a cardiopulmonary stress test, the actual milliliters of oxygen that are consumed by that patient per minute are measured. When we plug that number into a formula that adjusts for that patient's weight, we can determine their *actual* MET level.

We can also reasonably predict the *approximate* MET level of various activities, including different treadmill intensities, based upon data that has been collected from thousands of exercise tests and activity measurements from thousands of subjects.

For every 1.0 MET (which is consistent with being at rest), a person will use 3.5 ml of oxygen per minute for every kilogram of body weight. Therefore, if a person's body weight is 50 kilograms (approximately 110 pounds), at rest or at 1.0 MET, they use 3.5 ml of oxygen per minute multiplied by 50 kg. In other words, they use 175 ml of oxygen per minute under resting conditions, or at 1.0 MET.

If that 50 kg person exercises for 1 minute and uses 350 ml of oxygen, their body uses double the amount of oxygen as it did at rest. In other words, this person was exercising at twice the level of exertion as compared to resting conditions, or 2.0 METs.

Thankfully, we have averages for each treadmill level (intensity), so we don't have to figure it out every time. Instead, you can use the treadmill MET chart and age-predicted treadmill intensities I have provided for this purpose in chapter 6: Treadmill 101.

Subjective Measures of Exercise Intensity

Rating of Perceived Exertion (RPE) Scale

Named for its creator, Dr. Gunnar Borg, the Borg Scale or Rating of Perceived Exertion (RPE) Scale is simple to use and can be an invaluable tool for creating, monitoring, and modifying an exercise program. The original scale ranges from 6-20 and represents a subjective measure of how hard the person is working. A rating of 6 is equal to rest or very, very light exertion and a rating of 20 is equivalent to maximum exertion. Each number also corresponds to a description in words ranging from very, very light all the way to very, very hard.

Rating of Perceived Exertion (RPE) Scale	
6	
7	Very Very Light
8	
9	Very Light
10	
11	Fairly Light
12	
13	Somewhat Hard
14	
15	Hard
16	
17	Very Hard
18	
19	Very Very Hard
20	

Multiplying each number by 10 will give us an approximate heart rate range where 60 corresponds to the person's heart rate at rest and 200 corresponds to their heart rate at maximum exertion. There is also a modified version of this scale that ranges from 0-10, but in my opinion, the 6-20 scale works better and is the one we use at PWRC.

Most of your workout should take place in the "somewhat hard" range, increasing from *fairly light* at the beginning, working up to *somewhat hard* for most of the workout, and finally working *hard* at the peak, followed by a short cool-down period.

Perceived Dyspnea (Breathlessness) Scale

As compared to factors that can be observed by another person, like respiratory rate or increased work of breathing, dyspnea refers to a person's own internal perception of breathlessness. Like the RPE Scale, the Dyspnea (Breathlessness) Scale can be used to quantify the degree of shortness of breath a person is experiencing. This scale also ranges from 6-20, where a rating of 6 corresponds to none or very, very mild breathlessness and 20 corresponds to very, very strong breathlessness.

Perceived Dyspnea (Breathlessness) Scale	
6	
7	Very Very Mild
8	
9	Very Mild
10	
11	Fairly Mild
12	
13	Somewhat Strong
14	
15	Strong
16	
17	Very Strong
18	
19	Very Very Strong
20	

This information can then be correlated with more objective measures, like heart rate, blood pressure and oxygen saturation to determine safe and effective exercise parameters.

At PWRC, we continuously monitor our patients' heart rate and rhythm by EKG and their blood pressure and oxygen saturation are measured in five-minute intervals. We can also determine the percentage of your age- and gender-predicted maximum workload you're working at. That's what we mean by objective data.

As a point of reference, below are the *general* parameters that we use with our patients. This is assuming all things being equal, which they almost never are. As an example, if someone has known heart disease or pulmonary hypertension, we might make an adjustment to the below numbers to minimize the risk of a problem. Again, to be clear, these are *general* guidelines only. *Your* guidelines and limits should come from *your* physician.

Heart Rate: We will generally allow most of our patients to go up to a *maximum* heart rate of 200 minus their age (200-age). So, as an example, if we had an 80-year-old patient, we would allow him to go to a maximum heart rate of 120. The reason we use 200 instead of 220 is that it gives us a built-in 20 beat per minute safety zone, although most people don't reach that due to other factors like SOB or fatigue.

Blood Pressure: As far as blood pressure, if you are under eighty years of age, we will generally allow your systolic blood pressure to go to a *maximum* of 200 millimeters of mercury. If you are eighty years of age or older, we will generally allow your systolic blood pressure to go to a maximum of 180 millimeters of mercury. We generally try to keep diastolic pressures under 95 mm Hg.

Oxygen Saturation: As far as oxygen saturation goes, we try to keep our patients at 93% plus during exercise. In many cases, this means that we must use supplemental oxygen but in doing so, our patients are able to get a much better workout, as compared to room air and it is these more challenging workouts that lead to the greatest short- and long-term benefits.

Rating of Perceived Exertion (RPE): Again, when it comes to RPE, we generally want our patients to warm up in the "fairly light" to "somewhat hard" range, with most of the workout being in the "somewhat hard" range and "hard" range at the peak. Exercise in the "very light" or "very very light" range is too easy and exercise in the "very hard" to very very hard" range is too intense.

Perceived Dyspnea (Breathlessness): Similarly to RPE, when it comes to breathlessness, we generally want our patients to warm up in the "fairly mild" to "somewhat strong" range with most of the workout being in the "somewhat strong" range and "strong" range at the peak.

TIME (DURATION) OF EXERCISE

How much time you spend exercising is going to be dependent upon multiple factors and can vary from person to person, and sometimes even day to day. It will depend on your medical condition, your current level of fitness, and your degree of motivation (which, as you know, can be either your best friend or your worst enemy). And then there are those million and one other factors like going to work, picking up the grandkids from school, doctor's appointments, cooking and cleaning, etcetera, etcetera, etcetera. As John Lennon of the Beatles says: "Life is what happens while we're busy making other plans."

In an ideal world, we should exercise for a *minimum* of 20 minutes per day with a goal of 45 to 90 minutes per day. I know this is a big range, but it will make more sense later, when I give you sample workouts for 20 minutes, 30 minutes, 45 minutes, 60 minutes, and even a 90-minute workout for you exercise junkies.

In my experience with patients, the most effective workouts are between 30 and 60 minutes in duration with short rest breaks interspersed throughout the workout. If you can only tolerate 10 minutes of exercise (or less) at a time, you really need to be exercising two to three times per day. The good news is that there is evidence that suggests three 10-minute workouts per day are *almost* as effective as one 30-minute workout. Keep in mind that these workout times are in addition to all the other everyday activities you do.

TYPE OF EXERCISE

When we talk about the type of exercise, we are referring to the broad, general categories into which exercise can be divided. For the purposes of this book and my "typical" patient, I have included the five categories that we have found to be the most beneficial for people living with pulmonary disease. These five categories include breathing retraining, aerobic exercise, strength training, flexibility exercises, and balance training.

We will consider each of these categories from the perspective of both their *physiologic* impact on the body and their *functional* impact on the individual, during everyday activity. For example, when we talk about strength training, the physiological impact involves increasing the size of the muscles and the force with which they can contract.

When we talk about the functional impact, we are referring to the application of this force during everyday activities (e.g., getting up from a chair or lifting your grandchild). I will try to make this connection between physiologies and function whenever possible so that you have a clear understanding of how different exercises impact your everyday life. Then, you can decide which ones are most important *for you.*

Another key point is that whether it's in the physiology lab, at pulmonary rehab or in fitness magazines at the local supermarket, people often rigidly discuss and classify the types of exercise into distinct physiological and functional categories as if they some-how exist solely as independent entities and to the exclusion of all other categories. Most exercises and activities that we do involve a combination of two or more types of exercise.

In other words, even when you are doing what is traditionally considered to be aerobic exercise, you will still get secondary gains in strength, flexibility, and balance as well. Similarly, when doing strength training, you can also gain some aerobic and balance benefits, and finally, when you are doing stretching or flexibility exercises, you can also gain strength and aerobic benefits.

For example, walking is usually considered to be an aerobic activity, with elements of balance, strength, flexibility, and breath control required as well. However, when walking uphill or climbing stairs, a greater degree of muscle force is required making it more strength intensive. My point in mentioning this is to say that you will get at least some benefit in multiple areas during most physical activities.

Our goal is to create a program that incorporates each of these types of exercise that will give you the maximum benefit in the most areas with the least amount of time and effort. In other words, we want you to work smarter, not necessarily harder.

BREATHING RETRAINING

Breathing retraining includes diaphragmatic breathing, pursed-lip breathing, paced breathing, and recovery from shortness of breath. Although they are covered in Chapter 3, I wanted to mention them here in the context of exercise to keep things in their proper perspective (and chronologic order). These techniques provide you with greater breath control, which is why they are the first thing we teach our patients during their initial exercise session.

When you first begin learning and practicing these breathing methods, the techniques themselves are the actual exercises.

However, as you become more skilled in their application, you will use them as a *tool* that will allow you to do more vigorous exercise. It is this vigorous exercise that will ultimately decrease your shortness of breath, allowing you to walk more and potentially improving your lung function in the process. If you haven't done it yet, read about them, study them, practice them and use them both during your workouts and in your everyday life.

In Pulmonary Wellness Bootcamp, we address Breathing Retraining in every aspect of everything we do including Breathing Balance Flexibility Strength (BBFS), during the Walkabouts as well as during Meditation, Yoga, Tai Chi and Qigong.

AEROBIC EXERCISE

When people hear the words "aerobic exercise" or simply, "aerobics," their minds usually conjure up images of Jane Fonda or a room full of sweaty—I mean *glowing* women—in neon spandex jumping around, flailing their arms and legs to 80's disco music—and *a few* sweaty men. While that certainly qualifies, for the purposes of this chapter, I will define aerobic exercise as *any* activity that is cardiovascular in nature or what some people refer to simply as "cardio." In most cases, aerobic exercise involves rhythmic exercises that use large muscle groups and that can be sustained for *relatively* long periods of time. They will typically be lower in intensity than anaerobic exercise. Think tortoise, rather than hare, because if the intensity of the exercise is too great, you will be unable to sustain it long enough for it to be aerobic.

For anyone living with a cardiovascular or pulmonary disease, aerobic exercise is, by far, the single most important type of exercise. Aerobic exercise helps your body become more efficient at using oxygen and you, less short of breath. This can occur by:

1. Improving the mechanics of your respiratory system, allowing you to move air in and out more efficiently.
2. Improving the ability of your heart to pump blood to the lungs and throughout all the organs and tissues of the body.
3. Improving the efficiency with which your peripheral (or skeletal) muscles utilize oxygen, making them more efficient at extracting oxygen from the blood, and delivering waste products to the blood for removal.

In the context of our "supply and demand" conversation, aerobic exercise increases your body's oxygen supply while reducing its demand during physical activity, at rest and even while you sleep.

Examples of aerobic exercise include walking, jogging, cycling, swimming, and dancing, among others. If you're in the gym (or pulmonary rehab), cardio machines include the treadmill, stationary bicycle, upper body ergometer (UBE) and many others. To help you make the best choices for your own workout, I will take you through the pros and cons of each type and tell you what and why we do what we do with our patients.

Walking

Walking is one of the best possible exercises you can do, for several reasons. Most importantly, as human beings, walking is our primary mode of locomotion. If you cannot walk, this will severely limit your ability to get around and to participate in various activities of daily living, diminishing your overall quality of life. Walking can be done almost anywhere; indoors or outdoors and requires no special equipment other than comfortable clothing and a good pair of sneakers or walking shoes (and if you've seen some of the getups people work out in, you know that's not even entirely true).

Walking is multi-systemic and involves all exercise modes, not only enhancing aerobic capacity but also improving your strength, flexibility and balance and decreasing your shortness of breath in the process. It is also easily modifiable with respect to speed and duration, based on the individual.

Be sure to walk in a safe place like a gym, track, mall, or supermarket. Walk where the air is clean and avoid temperature extremes. If you are in a hot climate, walk early in the morning before the sun is at its strongest, or in the evening when the sun is starting to go down. If you live in a cold environment, walk indoors if the temperature is below approximately 36 degrees. Finally, if you are supposed to be using an assistive device like a walker or cane, please do. The same goes for any prescribed orthotics, where applicable.

Jogging/Running

Jogging and running have many of the same benefits of walking, but with a few caveats. The biggest difference between walking and jogging or running is that when you walk (even quickly), you always have at least one foot on the ground. When you jog or run there is at least a brief period during each stride (two) when both feet (and the rest of your body) are off the ground. As a result, there is a greater mechanical load every time your foot hits the floor. These factors increase the impact and potential stress on your body, particularly the musculoskeletal system (joints, tendons, ligaments), significantly increasing your chances of injury.

Both activities can range from fairly mild to very vigorous, so they can potentially generate even greater benefits with respect to aerobic capacity. However, this increased intensity also comes with some increased risk, which is why we usually recommend walking instead of jogging or running for most of our patients.

Treadmill

The treadmill is my single favorite piece of exercise equipment for many reasons. First, the treadmill is highly effective, mainly because its intensity can be easily adjusted with respect to speed and incline, making it a consistently measurable and "dose-controllable" activity.

Second, the treadmill provides mechanical assistance to ambulation (walking) by bringing your leg backward with each stride. This reduces the amount of force needed to overcome the resistance exerted on your body by the ground. For this reason, many people can do more on the treadmill than they can when walking, which ultimately helps you do more *off* the treadmill. As a point of reference, walking on a flat surface is equivalent to walking at approximately a 2% incline on a treadmill.

Finally, and this is so important, holding on to the arm rails closes the chain, allowing the muscles of the thorax and the entire upper body (pecs, lats, traps, serratus) to work in their reverse actions, assisting the diaphragm and allowing you to breathe easier.

I will address the treadmill in much greater detail as well as give you several sample workouts in *Chapter 8: Treadmill 101*. That's how valuable I think it is.

Bicycling

Riding a bicycle is another great exercise that most people can participate in (in one form or another). As they say, "it *is* like riding a bike." The bike is a relatively versatile and user-friendly piece of equipment. Its various parameters (body position, speed, and resistance) can all be modified based upon your cardio-respiratory fitness and any musculoskeletal limitations you may have, making it an effective workout tool for almost anybody.

Depending upon your body type and/or any physical or physiologic limitations you may have, you may find one bicycle to be more comfortable than another. As an example, because your back is supported, many people find the *recumbent bike* to be more comfortable and easier to use than an *upright bike*. However, this also makes the recumbent bike less physically (and metabolically) demanding than the upright bike.

Compared to the recumbent bike, there is also a strong postural component to the upright bike. In addition to the work of the lower body, the muscles of the thorax (chest, back and abdominals) must work harder to keep you upright, balancing anterior (front) and posterior (back) and left and right to prevent you from falling over. As a result, the upright bike is more physically (and metabolically) demanding than the recumbent bike. In other words, the upright bike requires more muscle activity, thereby increasing its value as an aerobic exercise.

Another consideration in choosing one bike versus another is the impact of body position on respiratory mechanics. When you're on the recumbent bike as compared to the upright, your knees come up a bit higher, bringing your thighs closer towards your upper body, compressing the abdominal and thoracic contents. As a result, the diaphragm has less room to contract (downward) and in fact, can be pushed upwards, further increasing the intra-abdominal and intra-thoracic pressures. These increased intra-abdominal and intra-thoracic pressures further compress the lungs, making it more difficult for you to take a deep breath. This is particularly true for overweight individuals, especially if they have a lot of soft tissue (fat) in the midsection.

Using a stationary bike indoors can eliminate the risks of outdoor cycling while still allowing you to develop both strength and aerobic capacity and if we set up a fan in front of you, you can still get that nice *wind-blowing-through-your-hair feeling* as you ride.

Elliptical Machine

Another one of my favorites, the elliptical machine is one of the most popular exercise machines on the market and for good reason. The elliptical offers a very effective full-body workout with many of the same aerobic benefits as jogging or walking with far less impact on the joints. Elliptical machines can be done using only the lower body (while holding on with the arms) or upper and lower body at the same time.

It is significantly more strenuous to do both arms and legs as opposed to just using your legs and requires a greater balance and coordination. Beginners should start using the lower body only for a less intense workout. As you feel more comfortable, you can add the arms, increasing the time and intensity as your fitness level improves. Be careful especially when getting on and off the machine.

Nu-Step

The Nu-Step is a semi-recumbent/recumbent cross trainer that combines forward and back arm motion (like the elliptical), with an up and down stepping motion in the legs (like a stepper), all in a seated or semi-reclining position. One of the greatest benefits of this type of design is that people of all fitness levels can use it, even if they are not capable of full weight bearing. The Nu-Step is extremely comfortable and consistently a favorite among patients.

Upper Body Ergometer (UBE) aka "Arm Bike"

The upper body ergometer (UBE) or "arm bike" is essentially a bicycle that you pedal with your arms. In most cases, you can pedal forwards or backward and the resistance can be adjusted to increase or decrease the tension, increasing or decreasing the intensity of the workout. The UBE is one of the best exercise machines on the market and almost always the first exercise we introduce our patients to in their initial session.

As human beings, we conduct most activities in front of us. As a result, the muscles on the front of the body are typically stronger (and consequently tighter) than those on the back, which are usually weaker (and looser). This muscle imbalance can lead to that round-shouldered, forward-bending posture that is so common as we age and even more so in people with respiratory disease.

For this reason, we usually have people pedal backward first, while they have the most energy to prioritize the back muscles. In this way, we strive to restore the body's natural muscle balance and upright posture. For patients with a significant forward bend (*kyphosis*), we may have them do the entire exercise backward. The

UBE is also very effective in relaxing the muscles of the upper body and the airways, increasing ribcage mobility, decreasing muscle tension, and allowing you to take a deeper breath.

Arm-R-Size/Arms-Up

Arm-R-Size is a series of 10-20 upper body movements that I believe I first learned at the UCSD pulmonary rehab program more than 20 years ago. We've been using it ever since and even added a few moves of our own. Essentially, these exercises simulate everyday activities, and each one can be done for 15-60 seconds (or more) in succession for a total exercise time of 5-15 minutes. One of the best things about this program is that it can be performed almost anywhere and doesn't require any special machines or equipment, making Arm-R-Size an invaluable addition to your overall workout or on its own.

For many people with pulmonary disease, upper body and particularly overhead (open chain) activities, are especially difficult; think washing your hair. These activities put the diaphragm and the rest of your respiratory muscles at a significant mechanical disadvantage for breathing, thereby causing you to become shorter of breath and your muscles (and you) to fatigue more quickly.

Arm-R-Size can help to prevent and reverse these effects increasing the strength and endurance of your upper body, improving the mechanics of your respiratory system, and desensitizing you to dyspnea, making your upper body muscles more efficient and you, less short of breath.

Swimming

Swimming is an excellent full-body, aerobic exercise for those that can do it. It has many of the same benefits of other aerobic exercise but creates less impact on the body due to the buoyancy of the water. However, swimming also requires a great deal of breath control and coordination, and the workout will vary depending upon which stroke you choose. Be aware that people whose respiratory triggers include strong odors or irritants may have increased sensitivity to the chemicals used in pools.

Water Aerobics

Water Aerobics combine various upper and lower body movements into a full-body aerobic workout. Working out in the water uses buoyancy to assist or resist the motion, reducing impact and increasing or decreasing the resistance depending on the muscles used. Again, be aware that people whose respiratory triggers include strong odors or irritants may have increased sensitivity to the chemicals used in pools.

Rowing Machine

A Rowing Machine replicates the act of rowing a boat (or more accurately, a racing shell). Stroke! Stroke! It's used in a seated position and is a full body exercise that combines a pushing (extension) motion with the legs and a pulling (flexion) motion with the arms. The rowing machine is an excellent workout for pulmonary patients and can be very beneficial in terms of posture. However, it may be difficult for people with limited joint motion, particularly in the lower back, hips, knees, and ankles.

In Pulmonary Wellness Bootcamp, we address Aerobic training in every aspect of everything we do including Breathing Balance Flexibility Strength (BBFS), during the Walkabouts as well as during Meditation, Yoga, Tai Chi and Qigong.

STRENGTH TRAINING

The goal of strength or resistance training is to increase the size (mass) of your muscles and the amount of force that they can generate. This is accomplished by exercising the muscles in a way that incrementally demands greater exertion, gradually increasing the resistance over time. This can be done using a variety of exercises, including free weights (barbells, dumbbells, wrist, and ankle weights), machines, therapeutic bands, isometric exercises, and activities that use your own body weight as resistance.

For pulmonary patients, we usually begin with aerobic exercise and gradually add strength training once you've improved your level of aerobic conditioning sufficiently. Generally, when you can do 15 minutes of arm exercises, 15 minutes of biking or Nu-Step and 25 minutes on the treadmill, we will then begin adding specific strength training exercises. However, as mentioned earlier, even an aerobic workout will help to improve your strength. For instance, if you are very weak, and you have been inactive, then going out for a walk—which is primarily an aerobic activity—will also increase your strength.

Strengthening exercises can be divided into compound and isolation movements. Compound movements are exercises that work several different muscle groups at the same time to achieve a specific motion or action, whereas isolation exercises focus on one muscle or muscle group at a time. As an example, the bench press is a compound movement whose primary muscle group is the chest or pectoral muscles, but they are assisted by the muscles on the front of the shoulder (anterior deltoid) and the triceps muscles on the back of the arms. The "pectoral fly" on the other hand, focuses on the chest muscles or pectorals alone, in isolation. Ideally, you would use a combination of compound and isolation movements depending upon your personal fitness goals.

In Pulmonary Wellness Bootcamp, we address Strength training in every aspect of everything we do including Breathing Balance Flexibility Strength (BBFS), during the Walkabouts as well as during Meditation, Yoga, Tai Chi and Qigong.

FLEXIBILITY EXERCISE

Flexibility or stretching exercises can increase your range of motion, decrease joint and muscle stiffness, and help prevent injury. While you may not need to be able to put your foot behind your head or twist yourself into a pretzel, flexibility is crucial to being able to breathe well and is essential to maintaining and improving your ability to perform a broad range of activities of daily living (ADL).

Due to poor respiratory mechanics and increased work of breathing, many people with pulmonary disease often develop muscle imbalances, particularly between the diaphragm and accessory muscles of breathing, as well as between anterior and posterior muscles of the body. Some muscles become tighter and shorter due to overuse, while others become weaker and overstretched. When this happens people may experience pain, particularly in the muscles of the neck, shoulders, back, chest and abdominals. This can further lead to skeletal adaptations of the spine and thorax.

Flexibility exercises can help correct or even prevent these imbalances, preserving diaphragmatic excursion and thoracic mobility and maximizing expansion of the lungs. In other words, flexibility exercises can help keep the respiratory muscles pliable, allowing the diaphragm to move freely and the chest and lungs to expand fully, decreasing the work of breathing.

Flexibility can also play an important role in everyday activities. For people living with a pulmonary condition, upper body, particularly overhead activities can be especially challenging. If you think back to our discussion of open chain vs. closed chain activities, you will recall that overhead (open chain) activities put the diaphragm at a significant mechanical disadvantage. In fact, people are often advised to avoid these activities altogether in the name of "energy conservation."

As an example, people are often told to avoid storing things on high shelves. However, if you don't use it, you lose it and avoiding these activities can lead to significantly decreased range of motion in the upper body, particularly, the shoulders. So, despite conventional wisdom, don't be so quick to avoid the activities that cause you discomfort.

Like aerobic exercise and strength training, there are several different types of flexibility or stretching exercises including static (stationary, including both active and passive), dynamic (moving), ballistic and isometric. Stretches can be used as part of your warm-up, mid-workout, or cool-down. For our purposes some combination of static and dynamic stretching would likely provide the greatest benefit while minimizing your risk of injury.

For those adventurous types who want to take your flexibility training to the next level you might consider alternative modalities such as Yoga, Pilates, Tai Chi or Qigong.

In Pulmonary Wellness Bootcamp, we address Flexibility training in every aspect of everything we do including Breathing Balance Flexibility Strength (BBFS), during the Walkabouts as well as during Meditation, Yoga, Tai Chi and Qigong.

BALANCE & STABILITY TRAINING

Balance and stability training should be an essential part of any exercise program. Good balance requires the interaction of the musculoskeletal system (strength and flexibility) and the neurologic system (coordination, proprioception, and sensation), among others. As we age, our balance and stability decrease, particularly if we have other conditions that diminish our strength, flexibility, and neurologic function.

Improving your balance enables you to maximize the benefits of your exercise routine and overall health and wellness program. More importantly, having good balance is essential for everyday activities.

Think about the role that balance plays in the following:

- Walking on uneven surfaces
- Walking up or down stairs
- Getting in and out of bed
- Getting into and out of the shower/bath
- Bending over to pick up something from the floor
- Overhead activities like getting something down from a shelf or changing a lightbulb
- Getting in and out of a car
- Getting up and down from the floor
- Being able to stand while riding the bus
- Line dancing or doing the conga at your niece's wedding!

There are a broad variety of balance and stability exercises, and some types may be more suitable for you than others. Balance activities can be divided into static (stationary) and dynamic (moving) activities. Some balance exercises can be performed at home, using only your own body, whereas others utilize specialized equipment such as stability balls, balance pads, foam rollers or wobble boards. In addition, there are a wealth of books, videos and classes that offer specific examples of individual or group balance exercises including alternative modalities such as Yoga, Pilates, Tai Chi or Qigong.

In Pulmonary Wellness Bootcamp, we address Balance training in every aspect of everything we do including Breathing Balance Flexibility Strength (BBFS), during the Walkabouts as well as during Meditation, Yoga, Tai Chi and Qigong.

FINAL NOTE:

As with any exercise program, please remember that safety is our number one priority. With that in mind, please check with your physician or health care provider before beginning any exercise program.

Chapter 12:

Treadmill 101 by Noah Greenspan, PT, DPT, CCS, EMT-B

"If you can't fly, then *run, if you can't run, then walk, if you can't walk, then crawl, but whatever you do you* have to keep moving forward." – Martin Luther King, Jr.

When it comes to the single best exercise for cardiopulmonary patients, the treadmill is in a class by itself. There are several important reasons for this. First and foremost, as human beings, we need to walk. Second, the treadmill is highly controllable and customizable, meaning that you can set very specific workout parameters for speed, incline, and consequently, workload or MET level. Finally, the treadmill physically assists your walking and provides mechanical support for your breathing, thereby allowing you to maximize your overall workout.

Patients often remark that walking on a treadmill is different and, in some ways, easier than walking outside or even from one room to the next. Notice that with each step forward, the treadmill moves your feet to the back of the belt, decreasing the resistance of the ground. As a point of reference, walking outside on a flat surface is the equivalent of walking at approximately a 2% incline on the treadmill.

Another factor is that when you fix your upper extremities by holding on to the handrails, the treadmill becomes a closed chain activity and divides the workload among four limbs instead of two. In addition, closing the chain greatly improves respiratory mechanics, allowing the muscles of your thorax; chest, back, shoulders to work in their reverse action, further assisting with ribcage elevation and overall thoracic expansion, allowing you to take a deeper breath.

Although we have touched on exercise multiple times throughout this book, I have not yet given you the specifics of treadmill exercise that you want and need. At this point, I would like to introduce some tools that will help you develop the absolute best treadmill protocol *for you* so that you can achieve the very best results within every workout.

As always, please do not begin any exercise program without clearing it with your doctor first, ideally after a comprehensive cardiac workup but at a minimum, some form of clinical exercise evaluation.

How Hard Should I Work Out?

When it comes to treadmill activity, patients often ask me some version of the following questions: (1) how hard should I work out, (2) what's more important: speed or incline, and (3) what's more important: time or distance. The answer is that they are all important and in fact, all directly related to and affected by one another. The longer you walk on the treadmill, the more mileage you will cover at a single speed. The faster you walk, the more mileage you will cover in the same amount of time.

However, when it comes to creating the most effective workout, that will not only produce the best results, but also have the greatest carryover to everyday life, MET Level (Measure of Exercise Tolerance or metabolic equivalent) is the most crucial (yet, frequently overlooked) factor. Also, when it comes to treadmill protocols and parameters, the MET is the great equalizer, allowing us to compare apples to apples and oranges to oranges.

As a quick review, one MET is equal to 3.5 mL of oxygen per kilogram of body weight per minute or the equivalent of your metabolic state at rest. This means that when you are at one met (think sitting quietly in a chair), your body consumes 3.5 milliliters of oxygen per minute for every kilogram (2.2 pounds) of your body weight. Activities at the two MET level would double your oxygen requirements to 7 mL of oxygen per kilogram of body weight per minute. Three METs would triple the workload and so on. You get the idea. As a point of reference, a workload of 1.1 METs to 2.9 METs is considered light, 3.0-5.9 METs is considered moderate and 6.0 METs or greater is considered vigorous activity.

Sadly, it is not only patients that are sometimes confused by this subject. Many healthcare professionals also struggle to understand how to create the most effective treadmill protocols and exercise goals for people with pulmonary conditions. In fact, if you read much of the classic literature pertaining to pulmonary rehabilitation, most people agree that patients feel less short of breath, can tolerate more activity, and have a greater sense of confidence and well-being. However, most claims fall short of promising improved pulmonary function.

In contrast, my colleagues and I *know* that you *can* improve pulmonary function *under the right conditions*. However, as opposed to the traditional low-intensity long-duration exercise used in more traditional programs, we have consistently found that it takes moderate and high-intensity exercise if you want to improve pulmonary function. For all these reasons, it is important for you to understand how to use MET level to your greatest advantage.

In this chapter, I will introduce you to two charts that we use at the Pulmonary Wellness & Rehabilitation Center: The Treadmill MET Chart and the American College of Sports Medicine's (ACSM) Age-Predicted Exercise Capacity (APEC Chart). Please do not be intimidated if they look complex at first. I promise after some explanation, they will make a lot of sense.

Treadmill MET Chart

The Treadmill MET Chart will tell you the MET Level for various combinations of speed and incline. The numbers across the bottom row of the chart represent speed in miles per hour (mph). The numbers in the first column on the left represent the percent incline (incline %). To determine the metabolic equivalent or MET Level, first find your speed along the bottom, and then match it up with the corresponding incline. MET level is found at the intersection of speed and incline.

TREADMILL MET CHART

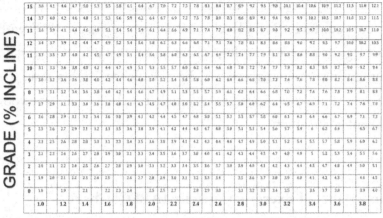

GRADE (% INCLINE)

SPEED IN MILES PER HOUR (MPH)

As an example, walking at 1.0 mph with no incline (0%) is equal to 1.8 METs. If we raise the speed to 1.6 mph, the MET level increases to 1.9 METs. If we then increase the incline to 3%, our MET level increases to 2.9 METs. You get the idea.

Here is another application. If you were to walk at 3.0 mph with a 0% incline, your level would be 3.3 METs. Now, three miles per hour may be too fast for many people (and too slow for others). However, if you were to lower that speed to 1.6 mph (approximately half), you could still reach that same 3.3 MET level by adding a 5% incline. Essentially, what this chart demonstrates is that there are many ways to accomplish the same MET level. This is an extremely valuable resource that will allow you to tailor your treadmill activity for maximum results, while individualizing the program to address and adapt to your own circumstances and abilities.

As an example, individuals with Spinal Stenosis, Osteoarthritis and other musculoskeletal conditions may have a harder time walking on a steep incline. In that case, you can increase the speed to achieve your target-MET level. Alternatively, if you are 4' 11" with short legs or have a neurological condition that affects your gait, maintaining a higher speed may be a challenge. In this case, you can walk at a slower speed with a higher incline to achieve your workout goal. Get it?

Age-Predicted Exercise Capacity (APEC) Chart

The ACSM's Age-Predicted Exercise Capacity (APEC) chart will tell you the percentage of exercise capacity predicted for a healthy person of your age and gender. To use this chart, first find your age on the left side. Then, take a ruler or sheet of paper and place it on your age. Then move the other side of the ruler to the MET level that you are working at (based on the treadmill MET chart). The point at which the ruler or paper intersects either the red line (for women) or the blue line (for men) represents the percentage of your age-predicted exercise capacity.

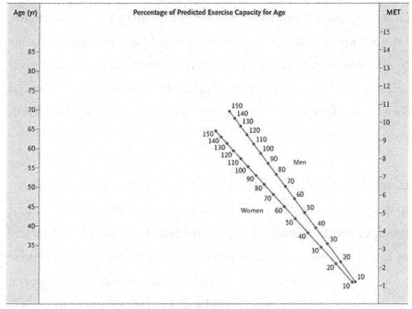

AMERICAN COLLEGE OF SPORTS MEDICINE (ACSM)
GUIDELINES FOR EXERCISE TESTING AND PRESCRIPTION

Here is another application. If you want to work out at a specific percentage of your age-predicted maximum, match up your age with the percentage of maximum that you would like to achieve and then extend the line to find out the appropriate MET level.

I encourage you to share these charts with your doctors and pulmonary rehab providers. They may or may not be aware of or practice this protocol but at The Pulmonary Wellness & Rehabilitation Center, we know that the MET counts for everything!

Creating a Treadmill Protocol

My goal with this chapter is to help you understand how to create the most effective and practical treadmill protocol *for you*.

However, while I can offer you general principles and strategies, I do not know your medical history and I have not had a chance to examine you or conduct any of my own testing to assess your abilities with respect to abilities and goals. Therefore, it is so crucial for you to clear any exercise suggestions you may see here with your physician.

In addition, if you have any cardiovascular risk factors or are prone to desaturation (among other conditions), you should not exercise unsupervised, at least in the beginning. I am also a realist and as much as I would love to recommend a personalized exercise program for you, I realize that many readers may be setting out on this journey alone, whether it be due to lack of access to a rehab facility, insurance, or other factors. Again, therefore it is crucial for you to speak with your doctor to ensure that you will be safe.

What if I don't have a Treadmill?

To be clear, I'm not saying that you can't get a good workout on a stationary bike or elliptical machine or even walking. These are all excellent alternatives. In fact, the best option is a cross training program in which you perform several different exercises within the same workout. But once again, if you want to choose the single best exercise that has the greatest chance of success, the treadmill would be my first choice, hands down.

Of course, if you do not have access to a treadmill, all is not lost. If that is your situation, then walk outside whenever possible. The

MET chart can still guide you in estimating your goals. Try speeding up or slowing down and find someplace with a varied terrain where you can increase the intensity of your workout using hills and slopes for inclines.

Other Considerations

1. **Clear all exercise with your doctor.** I cannot emphasize this enough. Ideally, I would like every patient to have a full physical examination as well as specific tests to assess cardiovascular risk such as a stress test with echocardiogram *at a minimum*. Under the right circumstances, exercise can be the best thing for you. Under the wrong circumstances, it can be the worst and as I have said before, when it comes to patient safety, I don't like surprises.

2. **If in doubt, refer to number 1.**

3. **Start slowly and progress gradually as tolerated.** Like Goldilocks, we like our workouts just right. However, it will always be better to err on the side of caution and underdo it rather than overdo it. Doing too much can increase your chances of an acute cardiac event or the development of an overuse injury, and sometimes you may not feel the full impact of the workout until several hours or days later. As I say to my patients: "everything will be done to your tolerance. Each time you come back and tell us that you felt well after the last session we will gradually increase your time and intensity."

4. **Think long-term and don't overdo it.** Let me put things in perspective for you. If you were to start off today walking on

the treadmill at 1.0 mph and added .1 mile per hour per week, in a year, you would be walking at 6.2 mph. If you were to start off today walking on the treadmill at 0% incline and added .5% per week, in a year, you would be walking at 26% incline. Now, I am not suggesting that you will be walking at 6.2 mph with a 26% incline. I'm just trying to say you don't have to do it all in the first week.

5. **Pay attention to warning signals.** As I say to my patients: "If at any time during the workout, you feel tired, dizzy, short of breath, chest pain or pressure, or you simply want to stop the workout, let me know right away." Since, I will not be with you, don't let me know. If you are unsure, stop. This is not an excuse *not* to exercise. I'm just saying that if you see any red flags, take them seriously.

6. **Push yourself whenever possible.** This may seem to contradict what I have just said in number 6. It doesn't. What I am saying is that if your life requires 5 METs, you can work out at 2 until the cows come home but your life will not be much different. Use the charts to figure out what speed, incline, and MET level you should be working at.

7. **Wear comfortable clothing and supportive sneakers or walking shoes.**

8. **Perform a gradual warm-up and cool-down.** The body doesn't like surprises. In other words, if you go from sitting in a chair to walking or running on the treadmill at your maximum capacity, your body can't tell the difference between that and getting chased by a bear and it could respond as such in the form of higher heart rates, and blood pressures, increased shortness of breath and decreased oxygen saturation. Another way to think

of your workout is like a flight. You want a nice gradual takeoff, a comfortable cruising altitude and a nice smooth landing.

9. **Don't stand still when the treadmill stops.** Most people's inclination is to stand on the treadmill for a few seconds when the belt stops. However, this can cause you to become light-headed or dizzy and in extreme cases, you could pass out. The reason for this is that when you are exercising, the heart is pumping blood to the body and the calf muscles return the blood from the lower part of the body to the heart. When you stand still, the heart is still pumping, and blood can pool in your lower extremities.

10. **Rely on your instruments.** Buy a pulse oximeter and blood pressure cuff so that you can measure your vital signs (heart rate, blood pressure and oxygen saturation) before, during, and after exercise. You cannot always go by how you feel. And again, when it comes to safety, we don't want to *assume*. We want to *know*.

11. **Do "the breathing."** Use controlled breathing techniques like abdominal breathing, pursed lip breathing and paced breath-ing. Time your breathing with your stepping. Breathe in, in, and blow- two, three, four (or whatever pattern works best for you).

12. **Use supplemental oxygen when necessary.** During exercise, we like our patients to be at a *minimum* oxygen saturation of 93% and we will use as much oxygen as necessary to keep them there. If you drop below 90%, you need oxygen. And given the choice, I would much rather give you more oxygen and allow you to do a bigger workout than not give it to you and have your workout be limited due to desaturation. Remember

that it is these big workouts that will allow for the greatest improvements.

13. **Take your short-acting bronchodilator ("rescue inhaler") 10-15 minutes before exercise.** Of course, you need to check with your physician on this one but again, our goal is the biggest workout possible, by any means necessary. So, if this will allow you to relax the airways, open the lungs and have a better workout, go for it!

14. **Exercise Testing and Prescription:** To be clear, all our patients come to us by physician referral. In addition, before we begin any exercise, we do our own treadmill testing using the Bensen Treadmill Protocol, developed by one of my former colleagues, Brooke Bensen. This allows us to determine exactly where a patient is at that moment and to set up a program that is going to be safe and the most effective.

15. **Sample Workouts:** On the Pulmonary Wellness Foundation's website, we have included many sample workouts based upon the protocols used at the Pulmonary Wellness & Rehabilitation Center. These are generic examples of low, high, and moderate intensity workouts. They are not specific recommendations for you or your situation. However, please feel free to share them with your healthcare team to help determine the appropriate starting point *for you.*

Here is the link:

https://pulmonarywellness.org/book-chapter-8-treadmill-101/

Chapter 13:

Pulmonary Nutrition

"The doctor of the future will no longer treat the human frame with drugs, but rather will cure and prevent disease with nutrition." – Thomas Edison

Written with gratitude to my Co-Author, Meredith Liss, MA, RDN, CDN, CDE, CLT

The subject of nutrition will almost invariably be included in any meaningful discussion of health and wellness. In the context of living well with a pulmonary disease, the conversation should be at least slightly (and in many cases, vastly) different than what most of us are used to hearing (and eating). In fact, sometimes recommendations made for the general population, particularly as they relate to cardiovascular diseases, diabetes, and obesity can be in direct conflict with the needs of people living with respiratory conditions.

Before I begin, please understand that this chapter is not a substitute for the medical advice of your physician or a personal consultation with a nutritionist. Instead, this chapter is a compilation of what I have come to believe are the most important principles as they relate to eating (and living) well with a pulmonary disease as well as information that will have the greatest impact on your respiratory system as well as your overall pulmonary wellness.

Like breathing itself, eating and nutrition are multi-factorial processes. The dynamics involved in what, why, and how people eat are many, diverse, and individualized; from physical and physiological, to intellectual, educational, and emotional, to financial and logistical, among many other factors.

As a result, we must first consider the impact that food has on breathing so you can begin to eat intelligently, systematically *and* in a manner that reasonably fits your lifestyle because if it doesn't, you *probably* won't do it and you *won't* be able to sustain it; in which case, these recommendations *won't* work. These strategies include thinking about and planning what happens before, during, and after individual meals, over the course of a given day or week *and* the weeks, months, or years to come.

Also, like breathing, the process of eating and nutrition can be divided into both mechanical and chemical processes. Therefore, I think it will be useful for you to have a basic understanding of the anatomy of the digestive system, particularly as it relates to the mechanics of breathing as well as the classifications of foods and their nutrients as they relate to our body's chemistry. By understanding these concepts, you'll be able to organize your eating behaviors to maximize your respiratory health and overall well-being.

I would bet that most people have a general (if not specific) idea of which foods are healthy and which foods are not, which foods will cause us to gain weight and which ones will help us lose weight; and which foods we should eat and which ones we should avoid, as well as which ones we should throw right in the trash.

Despite this basic knowledge, diet and nutrition remains one of the most difficult areas for people to implement and maintain successful and lasting changes in their lives. In the context of pulmonary disease, we also have the added responsibility of thinking about which foods (and other eating behaviors) will make us short of breath.

Nutrition is an extremely important, yet not extremely well understood component of living well with a pulmonary disease. While there is a tremendous wealth of knowledge about nutrition in the management of conditions like cardiovascular disease, diabetes, and obesity; far less is understood about the role of nutrition as it relates specifically to pulmonary health and wellness. This is particularly problematic because *what, when, why, and how we eat* all exert a tremendous impact on our health in general and our respiratory health and well-being.

As you probably know by now, I am completely biased in favor of exercise as the single greatest behavioral change you can implement to improve your health. However, nutrition comes in a very close second. In many cases (e.g., someone who is either severely overweight or severely underweight: two common scenarios in pulmonary disease), nutrition can even take center stage as your most important health priority.

Some nutritional issues will have a direct impact on our breathing. Some will be felt immediately, such as the increase in shortness of breath that you might experience after consuming a large meal (or a carbonated beverage or alcohol). Others will have more of an indirect or incidental effect, occurring over a longer period, such as the increased work of breathing that occurs following a 25-pound winter weight gain.

Conversely, not only do eating and nutrition impact your breathing, but breathing can also affect eating and nutrition. For example, being overweight, particularly around the midsection, can increase your shortness of breath. Now, with each breath, your body must lift those extra pounds around your waist. This can make activity more difficult, causing you to become more sedentary. As a result of this sedentary lifestyle, your body will burn fewer calories, causing you to gain even more weight (or at least making the weight more difficult to lose).

As another example, shortness of breath can decrease your appetite or impair your ability to prepare meals, making it a challenge to consume an adequate number of calories. Additionally, many people with respiratory disease are hyper-metabolic, meaning that they burn many times the normal number of calories than the average person. This accelerated metabolism is due to increased frequency (think respiratory rate) and work (think effort or intensity) of breathing.

As you can see, the processes of respiration and eating are intimately related and like many of the other cycles we have talked about, these processes can either work for or against you. My goal is to eliminate some of the mystery behind these relationships and improve your understanding of how you can best help yourself and your body get the most *out* of what you put *in*.

Steve Covey, author of *The Seven Habits of Highly Effective People*, has a great quote: "the main thing is to keep the main thing the main thing." As healthcare professionals, it is imperative for clinicians to spend an adequate amount of time learning about their patients. This includes understanding both the medical aspects of their disease, as well as getting to know them as human beings. We need to find out about their families, occupations, and personal habits (including what they eat) so we can ensure our patients' main thing remains the main thing.

As one example, in the context of Ultimate Pulmonary Wellness, many people don't get enough exercise. Others may be taking their medications incorrectly. For others, anxiety or depression may be their most paralyzing limitation. However, for many of our patients, nutrition is by far, their greatest challenge.

By meticulously getting to know each patient, we can focus on their most important priorities and not waste time on circumstances that do not apply to them. In most people's situations, nutrition should be included as one of the top priorities.

Basic Anatomy and Physiology of the Digestive System

The process of digestion begins in the mouth, where mastication (a fancy word for chewing) begins to *mechanically* break down food into smaller pieces. At the same time, enzymes in your saliva begin to *chemically* break down starches into simple sugars. From the mouth, food passes through the esophagus, which moves it into the stomach through a series of muscular contractions called *peristalsis*.

This step is very important and can often have a major impact on the respiratory system. The esophagus sits just behind the trachea, where the *epiglottis* prevents food from entering the trachea during swallowing. However, if the epiglottis is not functioning properly, food and other digestive contents (including stomach acid) can enter the trachea or even the smaller airways and the lungs.

When foreign materials enter the respiratory tract, they can trigger inflammation or obstruction in the pharynx, larynx, trachea, airways, and lungs. For a person who already has trouble breathing, this *reflux* can compound their respiratory problem by causing bronchoconstriction, bronchospasm, increased mucus production, or aspiration (when food or other substances are breathed directly into the airways or lungs), any of which can lead to further inflammation and/or infection.

From the esophagus, food travels through the lower esophageal sphincter into the stomach. The stomach is a hollow organ that churns the food with digestive enzymes and stomach acid. Food is further broken down into smaller and smaller particles and proteins are broken down into their component building blocks, amino acids.

From the stomach, food moves into the small intestine, which is made up of three parts: the duodenum, jejunum, and ileum. In the duodenum, food mixes with bile from the gallbladder (produced by the liver), neutralizing stomach acid and aiding in the digestion of fats. Enzymes from the pancreas also assist in the digestion of proteins, carbohydrates, and complex sugars. Nutrients are absorbed as they pass through the jejunum and ileum, including glucose (sugar), fatty acids, vitamins, and minerals. From the small intestine, waste products pass into the colon (large intestine), where water and minerals are reabsorbed into the blood, producing solid stool (debris and bacteria) for elimination through the rectum and anus.

The Relationship Between Eating and Breathing

Now, let's introduce a concept that is crucial to your understanding of how to maximize your nutritional status: the relationship between food, eating, digestion—and breathing. As I mentioned previously, some of these issues will directly impact your breathing, whereas others will have a more indirect effect. Some of these factors will be interconnected, and others will be stand-alone issues.

As I see it, the primary issues related to nutrition (food, eating, and digestion); as they affect and are affected by respiratory disease; can be broken down into several major categories. I will address each of them, one by one, and it will be up to you and your healthcare team to decide which issues are most important for you, and which ones may not apply to you at all.

Mechanical Aspects of Eating and Breathing

For the purposes of this discussion, it will be helpful if you think of the upper body as being divided into two separate compartments, like a suitcase. The upper compartment, called the thorax or thoracic cavity, houses the heart (within the mediastinum) and the lungs. The lower compartment, called the abdomen or abdominal cavity contains the stomach, liver, gallbladder, spleen, pancreas, intestines, kidneys, and adrenal glands. These two cavities are divided by the dome-shaped diaphragm: the primary muscle of inspiration.

The thoracic and abdominal cavities each have their own internal pressures called intra-thoracic and intra-abdominal pressures, respectively. However, even though they are separate entities, the intra-thoracic and intra-abdominal pressures are intimately related and can directly influence each other. If the pressure in one cavity rises, pressure in the other cavity can also rise (and vice versa).

Again, let's think back to our suitcase analogy with one side of the suitcase being the thorax and the other side, the abdomen. If you overstuff the thoracic side (as in the case of Emphysema)—the hyper-inflated (overfilled) lungs push downward, compressing the diaphragm and abdominal contents, increasing the pressure on the abdominal side. If you overstuff the abdominal side (as in the case of a large meal or constipation or bloating), the abdominal contents will push upward, resisting diaphragmatic excursion and lung expansion, increasing the pressure on the thoracic side.

Now, here's where things get interesting. The dome-shaped diaphragm lies between the thorax and the abdomen, sitting directly below the lungs in the thorax and above the stomach and intestines in the abdomen. When you take a breath, the diaphragm contracts in a downward direction, creating a negative pressure in the thorax. This negative pressure is what causes air to rush in, filling the lungs.

When the pressure in the abdominal cavity is increased (e.g., after you've eaten a large meal or become bloated with gas), there is increased resistance against the diaphragm's downward contraction. This puts the diaphragm at a significant mechanical disadvantage, making diaphragmatic contraction more difficult and causing you to feel shorter of breath.

In addition, the lungs can get pushed upwards and compressed, further reducing the amount of air that can be taken in with each breath. To make up for this reduced *volume* of air, you're now forced to breathe faster and more shallowly, working harder for each breath. If you recall from previous chapters, the more forcefully you try to breathe, the more airway narrowing, alveolar collapse and air trapping occurs, further increasing your work of breathing and shortness of breath.

Now, here is some further food for thought (pun intended). It doesn't matter if the obstruction is solid, liquid, or gas: full is full. This means that you must pay attention to the amount of solid food you ingest, the amount of liquid that you drink and the amount of gas you ingest (or produce). One way that this can occur is by accidentally swallowing air when you eat. However, if fullness and bloating are an issue for you, you should consider limiting carbonated beverages as well as solid foods and liquids known to cause gas.

Chemical Aspects of Eating and Breathing

It is important to realize that not all foods are created equal with respect to their chemical impact on breathing. Each type of food carries a specific chemical load. It is essential to realize that gram for gram; carbohydrate metabolism produces more carbon dioxide (CO_2) than the metabolism of either protein or fat. This is what makes high-carbohydrate meals particularly challenging for people with lung disease. Depending upon the size of the meal, the amount of carbohydrates, and the severity of your disease, results can vary from mild discomfort to acute respiratory distress.

The *Respiratory Quotient* (RQ) or *Respiratory Coefficient* is the ratio between the amount of carbon dioxide produced by the body and the amount of oxygen consumed during the metabolism of food. Carbohydrates have an RQ of 1.0. Proteins have an RQ of 0.8, and fat has an RQ of 0.7. In other words, if you eat 1 gram of protein, its RQ of 0.8 would produce only 80% of the carbon dioxide that would be produced by 1 gram of carbohydrate. If you eat 1 gram of fat, its RQ of 0.7 would produce only 70% of the carbon dioxide that would be produced by 1 gram of carbohydrate. In other words, eating a high carbohydrate meal can place a substantially greater workload on the respiratory system due to increased levels of CO_2 in the blood.

So, with every strand of spaghetti you eat (slight exaggeration), chemical receptors send a message to your brain that the CO2 level in your blood is high, which, as you may recall, is one of the primary stimuli of respiration. When the CO2 level in your blood rises, the brain sends out chemical impulses telling your respiratory system to breathe faster, deeper, and more forcefully, further increasing the work of breathing *and your SOB.*

Metabolism: Food as Fuel

Metabolism is a set of life-sustaining chemical processes and reactions that take place in every cell of our bodies. These include the process of digestion—the breaking down of foods into their component nutrients to release and supply energy and other essential substances to sustain all bodily structures and functions.

In the same way that a car needs to refuel every certain number of miles, we continually need to provide our bodies with the necessary nutrients based on the metabolic demands of our daily activities and individual energy use. At the most basic level, we eat to provide energy for our bodies to carry out all the functions of metabolism.

Nutritional Value of Foods

Besides the mechanical impact of food on breathing, it is also important to realize that not all foods are created equal. From a *nutritional* perspective, it may help to expand on our automobile analogy. In the same way that there are different grades of gasoline that can either enhance or hinder your vehicle's performance, the foods we eat can similarly affect our functioning. The higher the *quality* of the nutrients (food) we provide, the more efficiently they can be used and the higher "performance" you can expect from your body in the form of increased energy and activity tolerance and ultimately, reduced SOB.

What Should We Eat?

The *Harvard School of Public Health* created the *Healthy Eating Plate and the Healthy Eating Pyramid.* Instead of focusing only on the *quantity* we eat, Harvard's *Healthy Eating Plate* places equal—if not more—emphasis on food *quality.* In addition, the Healthy Eating Pyramid includes daily exercise and weight control in its core principles, two areas of particular importance for people living with a pulmonary disease.

According to the Harvard group, **half of your plate should be made up of fruits and vegetables.** A quarter of your plate should be made up of *whole* grains (not just any grains), **and the remaining quarter of your plate should be** *healthy* **protein. They also recommend using** *healthy* **fats and oils and drinking plenty of water as well as coffee or tea,** with no more than 1 to 2 servings of milk and dairy per day.

Please keep in mind that like everything else we discuss, there are caveats and exceptions to all recommendations or suggestions in this text and individual conditions must be applied. Many factors will determine what and how you should eat, including your age, gender, activity level, medical conditions(s), and medication(s). For this reason, rather than give you exact recommendations regarding specific foods and amounts, I'll present some general principles, which you can further explore with your physician, nutritionist, and other members of your healthcare team.

Here is a link to the Harvard HEP:

http://www.hsph.harvard.edu/nutritionsource/healthy-eating-plate

Fruits and Vegetables (½ Plate)

Fruits and vegetables are high in many essential nutrients and low in fat, sodium, and calories. They also have zero cholesterol. Eating a diet rich in fruits and vegetables is associated with improved pulmonary function and reduced risk of cardiovascular disease (e.g., hypertension, heart attack, and stroke), obesity, type 2 diabetes, osteoporosis and may also protect against certain types of cancers. Fruits and vegetables are also high in fiber, which lowers cholesterol and promotes healthy bowel function. No single fruit or vegetable contains all the nutrients that you need, so try to eat a wide variety to maximize your nutritional benefit.

Although Harvard's system suggests a combination of fruits and vegetables to comprise half of your plate, it is preferable—particularly for pulmonary patients—to focus on *non-starchy* (i.e., low-carb) vegetables, while grouping *starchy* (i.e., high-carb) vegetables with the grain portion of the plate.

Non-starchy vegetables include (but are not limited to) green leafy vegetables such as arugula, kale, spinach, Swiss chard, and watercress, as well as artichokes, asparagus, broccoli, Brussels sprouts, carrots, cauliflower, celery, cucumbers, eggplant, garlic, jicama, leeks, mushrooms, okra, onions, peppers, radishes, red cabbage, scallions, snow peas, tomatoes, yellow squash, and zucchini. Many of these can be eaten raw or cooked.

When we are talking about fruit, we mean fresh or frozen fruit, *not* juice or dried fruit as these are highly concentrated in carbs (sugars) and therefore, should be limited to two to three servings per day. Here are a few examples of a fruit serving: a small apple, ½ medium banana, ¾ cup of blackberries, ¾ cup of blueberries, 15 grapes, ½ mango, 1 cup of melon, small orange, peach, pear, ¾ cup of pineapple, 2 small plums, 1 cup of raspberries, and 1¼ cup of strawberries. The greater the variety you include, the healthier. Again, include but do not exceed two to three servings per day.

Whole Grains (¼ Plate)

Grains can be divided into whole grains and refined or processed grains. Whole grains contain the entire grain kernel (bran, germ, and endosperm) plus dietary fiber. Refined grains have been milled to remove the bran and germ, giving a finer texture, and prolonging their shelf life. However, the refining process also removes the dietary fiber, iron, and many B vitamins—in other words, most of the good stuff.

Whole grains are high in many essential nutrients, including dietary fiber, B vitamins (thiamin, riboflavin, niacin, and folic acid) and minerals (iron, magnesium, and selenium). Eating a diet rich in whole grains can lower cholesterol, reducing the risk of cardiovascular disease, stabilizing blood sugar, and lowering the risk of type 2 diabetes and obesity. A diet high in fiber also promotes healthy bowel function and can help prevent blood clots, a known cause of heart attack and stroke. Whenever possible, choose whole grains and whole grain products over processed grains for maximum nutritional benefit.

Whole grains include whole wheat (bread, cereal, or pasta), rye, barley, and bulgur, as well as gluten-free whole grains like buckwheat, millet, steel-cut oats, quinoa, and brown rice. Many products are made from refined grains including white flour, white bread, and white rice. "Enriched" grains have some of the B vitamins (thiamin, riboflavin, niacin, and folic acid) and iron added back but they are still not as healthy as whole grains.

When designating a quarter of your plate for whole grains, pulmonary patients should choose *either* a portion of whole grains *or* a portion of starchy vegetables, *not both*. For example, brown rice *or* whole-wheat pasta *or* potatoes *or* corn and *not* all of the above.

Healthy Protein (¼ Plate)

Protein can be obtained from both animal and plant sources and is crucial in the composition of bones, muscles, cartilage, skin, hair, and blood as well as enzymes, hormones, and vitamins, particularly the B vitamins. Proteins are also high in iron, which is critical in the transport of oxygen in the blood; magnesium, which is essential for building bones and releasing energy from the muscles; and zinc, which is important for fueling many biochemical reactions and boosting immune function.

While protein is essential for a healthy diet, some high-protein foods are healthier than others, so choose your protein sources wisely. Many foods that are high in protein (particularly protein from animal sources) also contain high amounts of sodium and/or saturated (unhealthy) fats. For example, although high in protein, red meat can contain high levels of both sodium and saturated fat. Processed meats (e.g., bacon, sausage, cold cuts) are notorious for being high in sodium and other chemicals often associated with inflammation and chronic diseases.

Therefore, it's preferable to choose healthy proteins like organic grass-fed beef (which is lower in saturated fat than conventional grain-fed beef), organic eggs, organic skinless poultry, and wild-caught fish; and limiting processed meat products.

When it comes to fish, be sure to include at least two meals per week of cold-water fatty fish such as salmon, sardines, herring, or mackerel for the anti-inflammatory benefit of the omega-3 fatty acids. You can also obtain protein from non-animal sources such as legumes (e.g., chickpeas, black beans, lentils), tofu, tempeh, seitan, unsalted nuts or seeds, and nut butters (e.g., peanut, cashew, almond).

Healthy Fats and Oils

Although fats and oils are often viewed as the enemy—leading to obesity, heart disease and a host of other health problems—this is not the case. In fact, healthy fats are cardio-*protective*, meaning that they protect the heart from atherosclerosis and coronary disease. Due to their high calorie content, healthy oils are particularly beneficial for patients who have a difficult time gaining or maintaining weight.

Fats can be classified into four main categories: saturated fat, polyunsaturated fat, monounsaturated fat, and trans-fat or trans-fatty acids.

Saturated fat can raise your blood cholesterol, a known risk factor for heart disease. Therefore, you want to limit the amount of saturated fat in your diet by eating less butter, high-fat cheeses, poultry skin, conventional grain-fed beef and any products made with palm kernel oil.

Polyunsaturated fats include both omega-6 fatty acids and omega-3 fatty acids. Both are essential for our diet. However, it is important to maintain the correct ratio of omega-6 fats to omega-3 fats.

The American diet contains excess omega-6 fatty acids because so many processed foods are made with vegetable oils derived from corn, cottonseed, safflower, sunflower, soybean, and "mixed vegetable oils."

We still need them in our diet, but when consumed *in excess*, omega-6 fats can trigger or increase inflammation. While this can be beneficial in times of illness or injury, inflammation is associated with increased risk of heart disease, diabetes, arthritis, osteoporosis, cancer, and respiratory disease. For all these reasons, it is recommended that we increase our intake of anti-inflammatory omega-3 fatty acids while limiting our intake of pro-inflammatory omega-6 fatty acids.

As I mentioned, the main sources of omega-3 fatty acids are cold-water fatty fish such as salmon, sardines, herring, or mackerel. If you are not a fish lover, you can get your omega-3 fats from land sources such as walnuts, ground flaxseeds, chia seeds, hemp seeds, canola oil and green leafy vegetables. You can also consider taking a supplement, which will be addressed later in this chapter.

When it comes to fats and oils, the bottom line is to enjoy foods rich in monounsaturated fats such as avocado, unsalted nuts and nut butters, seeds, olives, and olive oil.

Finally, trans-fats or *trans-fatty acids* are man-made fats. However, as of June 15, 2015, they have been taken off the FDA's Safe List and should be avoided at all costs. Trans-fats can be found in foods like margarine, commercially fried foods and baked goods made with either shortening or partially hydrogenated vegetable oils.

Dairy and Bone Health

Dairy products are a good source of calcium, vitamin D and potassium, and yogurt is an excellent source of probiotics, which are beneficial to digestive health. My gut feeling (pun intended) is that probiotics and the overall health of our gut also play a key role in reducing inflammation and boosting our immune function. However, according to the Harvard group, while calcium is important for building and maintaining healthy bones, there may be other sources that may be healthier and lead to fewer associated health risks. If you do plan to use dairy, replace whole milk, yogurt, and cheese with low-fat or fat-free products and limit their use to a maximum of one to two servings per day.

If you take or have taken steroids, you may be at increased risk for bone loss (i.e., osteopenia and osteoporosis). Therefore, it is important to pay attention to your intake of calcium *and* vitamin D (which aids in calcium absorption) and magnesium (to prevent any negative side effects of calcium).

Calcium-rich foods include dark green, leafy vegetables, canned sardines with bones, canned salmon, black-eyed peas, yogurt, cow's milk, cheese, calcium-fortified nut milks, and firm tofu. Adults ages 19-50 require 1000 mg per day. When women turn 50 and men turn 70, the requirement increases to 1200 mg daily.

Foods rich in vitamin D include salmon, tuna, sardines, eggs, fortified milk, and yogurt. Magnesium-rich foods include spinach, black beans, pumpkin seeds, almonds, cashews, soymilk, peanut butter, avocado, whole grain bread, brown rice, yogurt, salmon, and milk.

Dairy and Mucus Production

For as long as I can remember, people have been claiming that dairy products increase mucus production. I'm not going to make a case as to whether I think they do or don't. I will, however, remind you that everyone is different. So, if you feel that dairy products increase *your* mucus production, avoid them.

However, many people with COPD and other conditions in which mucus is a problem *can* tolerate at least some dairy. If you want to include dairy products in your diet, I wouldn't just accept the fact that you can't just because people have said so. This is particularly important for people who might be prone to calcium or vitamin D deficiency, including anyone who has been on steroids or who has additional protein needs due to muscle loss or weakness. Also, don't forget the probiotic benefits of yogurt for anyone who has taken antibiotics.

Not all dairy products are created equal. Most people find that skim products are easier to handle than whole dairy, but my suggestion would be to *try* them if you like them and see how you react (unless you are lactose intolerant or allergic). Also, start slow. Instead of drinking a quart of milk, try a sip or two or a couple of spoonsful of yogurt. If you tolerate this amount, you can gradually increase your "dosage."

Maintaining a Healthy Weight

Keeping your body at a healthy weight is extremely important and should be included in any discussion regarding the optimal management of pulmonary disease and health in general. This includes maintaining a normal weight versus being either over- or underweight as well as promoting good body composition (the percentages and ratios of body fat, lean muscle, bone, and water). As you probably realize, not all body weight is created equal.

To many, it may seem like being overweight or underweight are simply equal but opposite problems. If you're overweight, you simply need to eat less and get your butt off the couch and if you're underweight, I'm sure at some point, you've had to suffer the indignity of someone telling you how "lucky" you are because "you can eat anything you want and not gain weight."

However, *simply* losing or gaining weight is not actually simple at all. In fact, it can be extremely complex, especially in the context of pulmonary disease. In addition, sometimes your ability to lose or gain weight can be completely unrelated to anything you eat or don't eat or any exercise you do or don't do.

For example, if you've ever had to take steroids, you know prednisone can cause you to gain weight, particularly around the face and midsection. And for those of you who spend a good amount of your day gasping for air, you already know what it feels like to run a marathon—every day! While being overweight can have a significantly negative impact on your respiratory mechanics and your disease, being underweight is often a negative *consequence* of your disease.

If you have pulmonary disease and have either tried to lose weight or gain weight, you probably know that doing either one requires a sound (scientific) plan and a very healthy dose of willpower. Wouldn't it be great if those who are overweight could simply "donate" those extra pounds to those that are underweight? Of course, the situation is not always this cut and dried but let me explain further.

The Overweight Patient

As I mentioned earlier, being overweight can have a profoundly negative impact on your respiratory mechanics and increase your work of breathing. However, depending on the amount of excess weight, the problem can range from being a minor annoyance (if you are five or ten pounds overweight) to literally being the difference between life and death. I often see patients who are 25, 50, or even 100+ pounds overweight. If you are more than 25 pounds overweight, weight loss is unquestionably your highest priority and without a concentrated effort to lose the weight, it will be virtually impossible for you to achieve your full potential.

In addition to *how much* excess weight you are carrying, *where* your weight sits on your body can also have a major impact on breathing. Excess weight around the abdominal area will make breathing more difficult, forcing you to lift that excess weight with every breath. Think of it as weightlifting for your respiratory muscles. Is it any wonder why you're more fatigued?

Often, patients come to me with reports of increased shortness of breath even though their pulmonary function has remained stable. In fact, not much has changed at all except that they are now 15, 20, or 25 pounds heavier than the last time I saw them. Think of those extra pounds as two bowling balls pulling down on your thorax every time you need to take a breath. Being overweight contributes to increased shortness of breath, low energy, and decreased activity tolerance. Often, if patients can manage to lose the extra weight, their breathing problems improve dramatically.

When it comes to losing weight, exercise alone will *not* do it. Exercise is a major part of weight loss, but diet is at least equally if not more critical. In fact, I often tell my patients that they can out-eat any exercise program we give them. The healthiest strategies will include a combination of both healthier eating *and* increased physical activity.

The Underweight Patient

The underweight patient faces a completely different set of challenges. This is particularly challenging for PF and ILD patients and must be taken seriously. Due to increased work and frequency of breathing, the body's metabolic (and caloric) demand can increase dramatically. I don't believe the "10 times that of a normal person" that I've been hearing lately, but the difference in metabolism is significant compared to someone who is not constantly struggling to breathe. If weight loss progresses far enough and the person does not have sufficient fat stores, they will begin to burn muscle tissue for fuel. By the time the body reaches this point, the patient is often too weak to carry out even the simplest daily activities. Unfortunately, once you get to this point, their overall prognosis is poor if they cannot reverse this process.

Caloric Value of Food

From a *caloric* perspective, both protein and carbohydrates contain 4 calories per gram as compared to fats, which contain 9 calories per gram and alcohol contains 7 calories per gram. This makes calorie-dense (but healthy) fats a friend to the person trying to gain weight. *Do not* increase your alcohol intake as a weight-gain strategy unless you don't plan on getting much done. In addition to harming your liver, I'm sure you can see how this choice could lead to a whole host of other problems.

Now, let's take it one step further. A pound is made up of *approximately* 3500 calories. This means that to lose or gain one pound, you must either create a deficit of 3500 calories or a surplus of 3500 calories, respectively. In other words, if I consume 3500 fewer calories than I burn, I can reasonably expect to lose one pound. Conversely, if I consume 3500 calories more than I burn, I can expect to gain one pound.

Therefore, if your goal were to *lose* one pound per week, you'd need to create an average deficit of 500 calories per day (7 days per week x 500 calories per day = 3500 total calories). If your goal were to lose two pounds per week, you would need to create an average deficit of 1000 calories per day (7 x 1000 = 7000). This can be accomplished either by burning extra calories by increasing your exercise or activity, or by reducing your caloric intake by eating smaller portions or less calorie-dense foods. As I mentioned previously, a combination of both is more effective than either strategy alone.

Conversely, if your goal were to *gain* one pound per week, you'd need to create an average surplus of 500 calories per day. If your goal were to gain two pounds per week, you'd need to create an average surplus of 1000 calories per day. In the case of pulmonary patients, decreasing your activity is *not* recommended *at all*. Neither is increasing the size of your individual meals (which may not even be possible).

For all these reasons, gaining weight is often even more challenging for the underweight person than losing weight is for the overweight person. If you are underweight, it is crucial that you utilize strategies to increase your caloric intake by eating as much calorie-dense (but still healthy) food as you can in a way that will not significantly impair your breathing.

Many factors contribute to weight changes and there are no absolutes. So, instead of thinking of this as a hard and fast rule, use this mathematical approach to calories as a rough *guideline*. Make any necessary adjustments based on your own individual experiences and the recommendations of your healthcare team.

Hydration and Fluid Balance

Maintaining adequate hydration is important for everyone, but it is particularly crucial for people with pulmonary disease. Firstly, every part of the respiratory tract requires moisture to do its job effectively. In addition, hydration is important for thinning out your secretions, (mucus) keeping it moist, and allowing it to be expelled more easily. When we are dehydrated, our mucus becomes thicker and stickier, making it more difficult to expel and making you more prone to infection.

Many people have difficulty getting adequate hydration during the day for a variety of reasons. These can include anything from "I don't like water" to "the more I drink, the more I pee," among others. If you are not naturally a big water drinker, I know you're not going to go from drinking zero glasses of water to drinking the "recommended" 8-10 glasses per day. However, try to aim for a minimum of 4-5 glasses per day. A good indicator that you are getting enough fluids is that your urine is clear and colorless. People who are dehydrated often have highly concentrated, dark yellow or cloudy urine.

Also, when we talk about getting enough fluids, other drinks besides water count toward your overall fluid goal. So, again, if you are trying to gain weight, you should *avoid* drinking a lot of water since it fills you up *without* the benefit of having any calories. Instead, opt for calorie-containing beverages such as non-fat milk, a smoothie or low or zero-carb protein drink to maximize your caloric intake without increasing your carbohydrate load.

Also, don't drink before or during your meals. This can fill you up and prevent you from getting adequate calories and nutrition from your food. If lack of appetite or a feeling of fullness is an issue, you can get some of your fluids in the form of fruits, vegetables, and soups. Just be careful though because many soups contain a lot of sodium.

Conversely, people who are trying to lose weight should opt *only* for plain water or other non-caloric beverages whenever possible. You would be amazed at how many extra calories can be consumed in the form of caloric beverages. In addition, drinking water before or during a meal will make you feel fuller, allowing you to eat less and reducing your overall caloric intake.

IMPORTANT: Some people must be careful about consuming *too much* water. This includes people with renal (kidney) disease, heart failure and those taking diuretics, among others. While it is still important for these patients to remain hydrated, they should discuss their fluid requirements and restrictions with their physician.

Alcohol

When it comes to alcohol and cardiopulmonary disease, there are several considerations for you to be aware of. First, alcohol is a mild diuretic and increases the production of urine, making you pee more frequently. It also has a negative fluid impact, meaning if you drink one cup of alcohol, you lose more than one cup of fluid. Therefore, if you are going to drink alcohol, make sure that you are drinking extra (non-alcoholic) fluids to replace those flushed from your body to avoid becoming dehydrated (or too drunk).

Alcohol is a central nervous system depressant that lowers your heart rate and makes you breathe slower and more shallowly. Therefore, depending upon the condition of your lungs (and how much you drink), alcohol can make breathing more difficult, even causing respiratory distress or failure.

Also, alcohol can interact with your medications including prescription drugs, over the counter (OTC) drugs and nutritional supplements, potentially increasing the effects of some and making others less effective or not effective at all. Again, if you are going to drink alcohol, check with your doctor to determine if and how much is safe for you.

Finally, men and women metabolize alcohol differently. As a rule, men should limit alcohol to a *maximum* of two drinks per day, and women should consume no more than one drink per day. Now, before you start looking for that 64-ounce beer mug from college, one drink means 5 ounces of wine, 12 ounces of beer, or 1½ ounces of liquor. (Sorry, sports fans.)

Please understand that I am not trying to scare you, nor am I trying to convince you to become a teetotaler. I'm not. All I am saying is to use common sense. Be aware of the effects of alcohol on your body, and if you do decide to drink, moderation is the key.

Caffeine

Caffeine is a central nervous system *stimulant*, potentially increasing your heart rate, blood pressure and respiratory rate. This is particularly important for pulmonary patients because their hearts are often already working harder due to the increased work of breathing. In addition, certain classes of pulmonary medications—*beta-2 agonists*, can also be stimulants. Therefore, when used in combination, the two can make you feel jittery, anxious, or shorter of breath in addition to difficulty sleeping. Stimulants can also increase your risk of cardiac arrhythmias like tachycardia (fast heart rate) or atrial fibrillation, among others.

Sodium (Salt)

Unrefined salt provides two elements essential for life, sodium, and chloride. The American Heart Association recommends 1500 milligrams of sodium (or less) per day. However, while sodium is an essential nutrient, the average American often consumes more than double that amount and although seemingly harmless, most people don't understand the potential danger of an over-intake of salt.

Think back to our early discussions about the body maintaining equilibrium. This is true of the body's salinity (sodium level) as well. If you eat too much salt, your body will retain additional fluid to dilute the amount of sodium in your blood. This increased fluid retention can lead to an increase in blood pressure, causing the heart (particularly the left ventricle) to work harder. If left untreated over time, the ventricle can increase in overall size and thickness, requiring more oxygen to supply its increased muscle mass.

If the left ventricle cannot meet this excess demand (overload), fluid can back up into the pulmonary circulation, causing increased shortness of breath. This is known as left-sided or congestive heart failure. Left unchecked, blood can continue backwards through the pulmonary circulation to the right side of the heart, eventually pooling in the lower extremities (pedal edema). This is what is known as right-sided heart failure. The bottom line is "easy on the salt!"

Instead of salt, use onions, garlic, herbs, spices, citrus juices, and vinegars to flavor your food. Experiment with basil, curry, dill, oregano, paprika, parsley, rosemary, sage, thyme, turmeric, and other salt-free flavorings.

Minimize your use of high sodium foods such as smoked, cured, salted, or canned meat, fish, or poultry (including bacon, cold cuts, ham, hot dogs, sausage, caviar, and anchovies). Choose fresh or frozen vegetables instead of canned (high in salt). Drain and rinse canned beans and choose low-sodium versions of canned soups. Also, choose unsalted nuts and seeds.

Food Allergies and Sensitivities

Often, people with respiratory disease also suffer from food or other allergies, which can have a negative impact on both the upper and lower respiratory tracts as well as your body's overall inflammatory and immune responses. Food allergies occur when your body's immune system overreacts to a food or substance that it *mistakenly* perceives as a threat.

Food allergies can range from mild to life threatening (anaphylaxis). The most common manifestation of food allergies is *chronic rhinitis* or inflammation of the mucus membranes in the nose, but food allergies can also impact the respiratory system in the form of shortness of breath, cough, tightness in the throat or difficulty swallowing, wheezing, airway obstruction and swelling of the lips, face, and tongue.

You may be surprised to hear that 90% of all dietary allergies are caused by 8 foods. These include eggs, milk and dairy products, peanuts, tree nuts (pecans, walnuts, almonds), fish, shellfish (shrimp, crab, lobster), wheat or gluten and soy. People with specific food allergies may also react to similar or related foods. The severity of symptoms is generally associated with the amount of the allergen ingested, but as a rule, it is best to eliminate the offender from your diet completely.

Gas and Bloating

Excessive gas and bloating can also create problems for people with respiratory disease. Again, think about everything that takes up space in your stomach, increasing the intra-abdominal pressure. Remember, your body doesn't care if this increased pressure is due to solid, liquid or gas. If gas or bloating is a problem for you, consider limiting or avoiding gas-producing foods and carbonated beverages. As an alternative, you can try using an enzyme-based, gas-reducing food additive like Beano.

Fiber

Fiber is a form of carbohydrate that regulates blood sugar, promotes the passage of food through your system and may help prevent many chronic diseases. Constipation can increase intra-abdominal and intra-thoracic pressures, making breathing more difficult. We should try to eat 20 to 30 grams of fiber per day in the form of whole grains, fruits and vegetables and beans. If gas and bloating are a problem for you, low-FODMAP, fiber-rich foods include oatmeal, oat bran, brown rice, rice bran, chia seeds, flax seeds, strawberries, blueberries, oranges, spinach, and quinoa.

Gastroesophageal Reflux Disease (GERD)

Often, people with respiratory disease also suffer from another condition called Gastro-Esophageal Reflux Disease (GERD). Many are not even aware of it (silent reflux), but GERD can cause, trigger, or worsen their respiratory condition (and vice versa). Often, once GERD is discovered and treated, their respiratory condition improves as well.

GERD is caused when acid backs up from the stomach through the lower esophageal sphincter, damaging the esophagus, throat, and possibly, the airways and lungs. While the most common symptom of acid reflux is heartburn, GERD can also cause a sore throat, bitter taste in the throat and mouth, chest discomfort (non-cardiac) and abdominal pain, as well as many "respiratory" symptoms such as coughing, wheezing, and shortness of breath.

The exact cause of acid reflux and GERD is unknown, but several factors contribute to or exacerbate the problem, including obesity, diet (particularly fried, fatty, spicy, and acidic foods like citrus and tomatoes), caffeinated beverages and chocolate and mint flavorings. Drinking alcohol or cigarette smoking can also exacerbate the problem, as can certain medications including antihistamines, calcium-channel blockers, nitrates, and theophylline, sometimes used to treat pulmonary disease. Consuming large meals or eating close to bedtime can also contribute to GERD. Finally, GERD can result from other medical conditions like hiatal hernia, pregnancy, rapid weight gain and diabetes.

Lifestyle modifications for people suffering from GERD include weight loss, dietary modifications (e.g., avoiding known triggers, eating smaller and more frequent meals, and not eating or drinking close to bedtime). Quitting smoking and minimizing alcohol intake are also recommended.

Elevating the head of your bed by 6-12 inches (or sleeping with a wedge) can help reduce symptoms. Pharmaceutical and surgical options are also available but are beyond the scope of this text and should be discussed with your physician.

Nutritional Supplements

First and foremost, it is important to understand that vitamins and minerals are best utilized if you get them as part of a healthy, balanced diet. Be sure to include foods rich in antioxidants such as vitamin C (red pepper, green pepper, papaya, strawberries, broccoli, oranges, cantaloupe), vitamin E (sunflower seeds, almonds, hazelnuts), selenium (Brazil nuts, tuna, sardines, salmon, sunflower seeds), and carotenoids (carrots, sweet potatoes, red peppers, spinach, cantaloupe, kale, collard greens, mango, butternut squash).

If you have difficulty getting all your vitamins from food, you may want a little extra insurance. Choose a complete, *age-adjusted* multivitamin that contains 100% of what you need but not more and take it either once daily or every other day. Avoid the MEGA-vitamins as too much of a good thing will either wind up in your toilet bowl in the form of very expensive urine, or worse, cause harm. Speak to your physician or nutritionist about the right type and dose of supplements for you.

As we discussed, calcium, vitamin D and magnesium are important for bone health, especially if you are at increased risk for osteoporosis or have been on steroids. Again, do not go above the recommended daily dose and when taking a calcium supplement, be sure that it also contains vitamin D and magnesium. If your vitamin D level is low (get it checked!), you can supplement with additional vitamin D3.

Finally, a high-quality omega-3 fish oil supplement is beneficial due to its cardio-protective and overall anti-inflammatory properties. Choose a fish oil supplement with a decent dose of both eicosatetraenoic acid (EPA) and docosahexaenoic acid (DHA). Don't be fooled by supplements that boast 1000 mg of fish oil; you need to make sure you are getting actual DHA, and EPA as other oils are sometimes included in the 1000 mg of "fish oil." Compare labels and choose supplements with high amounts of these two beneficial fatty acids.

For herbal and homeopathic remedies, I strongly suggest carefully evaluating them on a case-by-case basis with your doctor, nutritionist, or pharmacist, especially as they may affect your medical condition and medications.

Tips for Eating for Pulmonary Patients

- Avoid large meals. Instead of 2-3 large meals, eat 5-6 smaller "*feedings*" per day. In other words, eat frequently (roughly every 2-4 hours, depending on your goals) but in small quantities so that the food you eat doesn't take up all your available breathing space.
- If decreased appetite is an issue or you are trying to gain weight, drink at the end of your meal as opposed to before or during.
- If you are trying to lose weight, drink water before and during your meal.
- During the meal, pace yourself and use pursed-lip breathing.
- If shortness of breath is an issue, use your rescue inhaler 15 minutes before eating.
- If you use supplemental oxygen, wear it while you eat.
- If secretions are a problem, clear your airway before eating.
- Keep a food diary to monitor the impact of different foods on your breathing and energy levels.
- Eat mindfully, not mindlessly.

Keeping a Food Diary

Write everything down that you eat and drink including time, how much you ate and how you felt afterwards. Take note of food's impact on your shortness of breath and energy levels and record those in your diary. Observe how your body reacts to different foods with respect to type, amount, and timing. Keeping a diary will also make it easier for your physician or nutritionist to understand your needs and offer the most effective advice.

I often say: "if you want to change your life, you have to change your life." That is, if you want to see significant results, you need to make a significant change. Changes that don't require any discipline will not lead to the changes that you want. A coordinated effort and a little willpower will help you find and stick with a nutrition program that fits *your* lifestyle and *your* health needs.

Chapter 14:

Emotional Health & Well-being by Grace McKeown, John LaJeunesse & Charlene Marshall

Pulmonary fibrosis elicits several emotional responses, because it threatens the very thing most people take for granted... *our ability to breathe!*

In this section, we explore various emotional responses that might occur following the diagnosis of pulmonary fibrosis. We hope that your emotional and mental health can be spared a little from the challenges we encountered following our own diagnoses, and that our experiences bring you some comfort. We aren't supposed to *know how* to cope with a life-threatening diagnosis, and we acknowledge that there is no how-to guide to help us.

When given the diagnosis of an interstitial lung disease (ILD) such as PF, we have already lived in a world where we've experienced various stressors and strains that influence our ability to cope with adversity. We often come from vastly different life experiences by the time we become part of the ILD community, post-diagnosis. These experiences will inevitably influence our emotional responses to a diagnosis like PF, and these responses will vary widely.

Some important factors to take into consideration which might affect one's emotional response to PF, is their diagnostic experience, age and like we mentioned already, previous life experiences.

Regardless of whether your diagnosis of PF is abrupt or occurs following a prolonged period seeking answers; how you feel is both valid and understandable. Charlene Marshall is one of the authors of this book, and as an IPF patient who is privileged to interact with many other patients, including those who are newly diagnosed, she hears regularly how varied people's responses are to their diagnosis. Charlene shares this about her own IPF diagnosis in 2016:

"Personally, I (Charlene) felt as though I was regurgitating someone else's sad story; I didn't know anything about IPF and couldn't comprehend that my young and otherwise healthy body was dealing with a terminal illness. Initially, I believe my coping strategy was avoidance and I really didn't think about what life would be like post-diagnosis."

Charlene further shares that her mental health, prior to her diagnosis, was stable and that she had previously developed effective coping strategies. This helped her tremendously when the reality of having a life-threatening lung disease like IPF finally started to sink in. Charlene recognizes that not everyone has developed effective coping skills, which further complicates how some may respond to a diagnosis like PF, especially in addition to other stressors in a patient's life.

Before diving into this chapter further, we want to re-introduce you to its authors.

John is the most recently diagnosed of all the authors, although there have been many stressful parts of his life that he is also coping with. He also has been a mentor to his brother who has an even more recent diagnosis of PF.

Charlene is the baby; she is the youngest of the group in both chronological age and at diagnosis. She is an active patient and advocate, and you may know her work with Pulmonary Fibrosis News. She was instrumental, alongside Noah Greenspan, in formulating this group.

Grace, that's me; the "oldie" of the group being 80 years old and having PF the longest, as my diagnosis was in 2006. You may have gathered more about us from the first chapter, introducing us and the other contributors to this book.

Emotional scars can be traced back to a variety of stressors that have occurred in our lives. Let's look at some commonalities of how people may respond to life-threatening news and consider some strategies to reduce the impact of stress on ourselves and our loved ones. *Did you know that a diagnosis of a life-threatening illness can elicit responses likened to grief, even though a death hasn't occurred?*

When John was diagnosed with PF, his spouse felt as though she had been cheated somehow because the diagnosis was unsuspecting. When this happens, there is an-almost deafening silence amongst your loved ones. If they seem distant or impartial, it might be because they've already surrendered their heart to the loss of you. Since we all come with various life experiences, they may have already suffered losses which could be triggering, so please don't turn your back on them.

One of the original grief response models by Elizabeth Kubler-Ross, has been adapted in recent years, but her work has undoubtedly shaped people's understanding of how we respond to death, chronic illness, or life-threatening news. Her underlying message is that not everyone experiences each stage or corresponding emotional response in the same order, and the time spent in each is varied and non-linear, and how you feel today might drastically differ from tomorrow.

This has been my (Grace) experience, and my responses have repeated themselves at various stages of this disease. At first, it felt disappointing that I had not moved on, but now it feels more like a relief. *"I have been here before"* becomes an inner message that gives me strength.

For this chapter, we'll use the Kubler-Ross model to outline the stages someone might experience in response to their diagnosis. Those stages are denial, anger, bargaining, depression, and acceptance. Since the original publication of Ross' work, some modifications have been suggested, including shock, and we add them here where relevant.

As you may have previously experienced throughout your life, grief can consume you physically and emotionally. Grief in response to a chronic illness is a complex process, and we see it at various times when changes in the illness trajectory occur, such as progression of the disease. Before we get into the original stages of Ross' model, we as patients, face the shock of a PF diagnosis.

SHOCK

It likely won't come as a surprise to you that shock is one of the first emotional responses that many people experience. In addition to shock, many of us feel fear, dread, and panic. Our cough or shortness of breath has been a nuisance over the years and none of the usual remedies have helped. Eventually, after being pushed by family you visit a doctor, which results in a prescribed remedy. It's a bit of a pain when the remedy doesn't make any difference. Sometimes even the third or fourth prescription doesn't even help and the cough returns. An x-ray seems like the next logical step, but it can be alarming to then have a series of investigations set in motion based on those x-ray results. These tests likely include bloodwork, pulmonary function tests, cardiac diagnostics, and a high-resolution CT scan. Although alarming, it can also feel reassuring because a solution will emerge, and all this investigation can only be useful in our quest for answers.

Even throughout the investigative process, patient's experience a range of emotions and we haven't even received a diagnosis yet. There is likely to be some anxiety, often unspoken, about what these symptoms could be, like cancer. When no cancer is found, it's normal to feel relieved. Phew, now that you know it isn't cancer, you feel like you can breathe again, metaphorically speaking of course! However, the emotional challenges come from the eventual diagnosis, and it's perplexing that all these investigative tests result in a diagnosis that does not have a cure, or even remedies to help.

Unfortunately, that's the reality of a progressive illness such as PF, and despite the physician's efforts, it's not easy to deliver this diagnosis to a patient or their family. In Charlene's diagnostic experience, she remembers fixating on the following words: "life-threatening," "progressive," "lung failure," and "oxygen." She couldn't focus on anything else, no matter how many ways the specialist tried to soften the diagnosis.

All suffice to say, a diagnosis of PF would be a shock to anyone, whether the process for you mirrored the scenario above or it was like the experience told by other authors of this book. How we respond to shock depends on previous experiences in our lives.

I (Grace), for example, was quite proud of the fact that I don't have a panic button, so others expected that I would be able to cope with this and I did. I got on with my life and saw no reason not to continue with my plans to embrace permaculture. I planned to spend my time between England, where I could be part of my grandchildren's life, and Spain, where I could contribute to community development initiatives and ecological protection of the environment. It was not in my plans to let PF get in the way of these desires! It may have been useful to accept that changes to my lung function would happen, and in hindsight, I question whether part of my coping could be explained in the grief model as denial.

DENIAL

In the early stages of grief, often felt when diagnosed with a chronic illness, it is counterproductive to deny the truth of the disease, but this is the reality of many patients' response. Denial, however, is a natural response and can be the proverbial "breathing space" we might need to come to terms with our diagnosis. Denial forces us to delay some decisions that will have to be made and shields us from the sorrows and regrets that we are sensing but not yet ready to look at. This can be a particularly difficult time for caregivers, especially if they are feeling ready to face the disease head-on and the patient is in denial. See chapter 3 on caregiving for more information.

ANGER

Where denial as a short-term emotional response can give time for us to find a way to cope with some of the changes; anger can act as a mask for other emotions building inside patients newly diagnosed with PF. However, anger can be the stimulus that drives us to learn more about PF and how to cope with it. It was my (Grace) anger about the lack of information provided by my clinicians that drove my original research into the disease. I didn't recognize this as anger at the time, simply because I do not view myself as an angry person.

Like all responses in Ross' model, anger is not an emotion felt by everyone. It's hard not to feel resentful or angry with others who have made poor health choices throughout the years, such as those who smoke but remain 'fit and healthy' and yet for us, walking a couple of feet is challenging. Anger can also force self-reflection and help us turn inward and explore what might have contributed to our diagnosis (though, it's important not to blame yourself). Self-reflection allows us to think about things differently and examine: *what can now be changed in our lives to help preserve our respiratory health?*

When experiencing anger, it doesn't feel possible that it's potentially be a positive thing for us but be patient with yourself or your loved ones; there is a lot to be angry about and it's important to process those things. For example, the way life was "supposed to go" is inevitably going to be different for patients, and as a caregiver, you may not have expected this role and resent it.

"Why?" is a question that has no answer and can make us so angry. Finding ways to disperse that anger by journaling, talking to a friend who will just let us be angry, expressing it out loud to oneself and finding a safe physical outlet are all useful strategies for dealing with anger. I (John) have managed to come to terms with my anger by deeply pondering the impact my diagnosis has had on my family. I try not to be as hard on myself anymore and now I lean on my family when I'm feeling low. I still have good and bad days but, I'm able to remember that just as I care about my longevity, so do my significant others. I try to be positive for myself but mostly for them.

BARGAINING

Just as we can't bring a loved one back from the dead, we also can't turn back the clock to our pre-ILD life. For people who are religious and believe in the power of prayer, it may feel beneficial to increase the time praying. As an example, bargaining can mean returning to church for some people and with that, an increase in support.

Wanting to bargain to influence the outcome of life with an ILD is not restricted to a religion. We may tell ourselves that there are always exceptions to a poor prognosis. For example, if good nutrition hasn't been taken seriously up to the point of diagnosis, committing to a healthy lifestyle might become a bargain with the expectation of a different outcome. Further, building a support network through a social community for example, or embarking on a healthy eating journey will have a positive influence on our general well-being, which may be a bargain worth exploring simply for the benefits it will provide. If the goal of bargaining however is to eradicate our diagnosis of PF through healthier choices, which unfortunately won't happen, the emotional response to bargaining can turn to deep sadness about the reality we are facing.

DEPRESSION

This time of deep sadness can be a real challenge for anyone who has not previously had experience with depression. It can feel as though depression takes over one's life and is immobilizing.

Depression can make decisions feel impossible and thinking foggy and disjointed. As a temporary stage when dealing with the roller coaster of emotions involved in a progressive illness, depression is very common and can even be beneficial as we face different stages of the illness.

I (Grace) did get very down recently, even after living with PF for years. My pulmonary consultant appeared to be writing me off from any further intervention and it was clear that a decision had been made that I was in the end stage of this illness. The problem was that it was not being talked about openly. I oscillated between fear of what appeared to be thought about me and disappointment that the work that I had put into building the relationship with my clinicians seemed of no value.

As a result, sadness made me stop once again, though I knew I had been here before. I also was feeling scared. Again, I felt the despair that PF was catching up with me and that I was approaching death. I felt exhausted, and my shortness of breath was the most debilitating it had been for years. Expressing how I felt to family and friends was what enabled me to move through this. I also shared how I felt via email to my consultant and made him aware of the negative response that can be felt by patients regarding poorly presented information.

ACCEPTANCE

This stage sounds almost idyllic and feels like it guarantees happiness, but that is not it's intention. In some ways, acceptance is the starting point of *living* "life with PF;" accepting life with a lung disease as opposed to clinging to life before the diagnosis. For some, acceptance may be a stage that comes early in the journey, whereas for others, reaching this stage is very difficult. It means that we look toward a future despite all its unknowns.

Acceptance can also be a stage of change; the start of focusing on well-being and prioritizing our mental health, for example. Acceptance can move us to do incredible things, despite the adversities we are facing. Despite living with PF, all the authors of this book have accepted our disease, albeit begrudgingly as no one wants to have PF, and committed to taking our experience and writing about it to help others.

STRESS

Stress is how our bodies react to the demands we face in the world. The stress of losing one's ability to breathe can make other stresses seem trivial by comparison, but it's important to still recognize and acknowledge those stressors as having an impact on us. Stress can also lead to feeling anxious, concerned, despondent, depressed and a whole variety of what-are-considered to be negative emotional responses. Navigating emotions connected to a life-threatening lung disease is unknown terrain for all of us.

Feeling anxious is a common response to stress and something most of us are aware of, however stress is not all bad. The fancy name for stress that elicits positive responses is eustress; it can be a motivator and even contribute to a "feel good" sensation when we let it. Remembering that point; *when we let it*; is very important and reminds us of what we do have in our control, especially when we don't feel in control.

I (Grace) can find it stressful to motivate myself to get out for my walk, for example. I live in a southwest city in the UK, and it means a car ride to the open countryside. I often feel exhausted just preparing an adequate supply of oxygen to take with me, dressing for the weather and getting into the car. On good days, these tasks seem simple, but on bad days it can feel like trying to climb a cliff face without a rope. I talk to myself during this time and remind myself of some positives or that I have felt this way before but came through this stress before.

The positive feeling I get from an outing is not only the satisfaction that I had walked, but physically I feel better too. This is the dopamine response in my brain that's been stimulated I realize from some of my research and for me, just feeling better is good enough. In fact, this 'feel good factor' can then set off a chain of positive events

There is often anxiety around the "what ifs" as well. When stress elicits negative emotional responses, including anxiety and depression, the effects can be felt to varying degrees. For example, stress, anxiety, or depression may show up in physical, mental, or behavioral forms so it is useful to address them when symptoms appear.

In the chapter on oxygen, Linda has outlined the use of a pulse oximeter to check oxygen saturation. Simply seeing that our oxygen levels are ok is comforting when we are short of breath (SOB), even though we know that SOB does not always correlate to an oxygen drop. Seeing our oxygen saturation helps us realize that anxiety might be playing a part in our SOB. The fear or general anxiety that other organs in our bodies are deteriorating is very understandable. When emotional tension and stress come are present, our bodies can manifest a variety of changes identified as physical, emotional, or behavioral.

PHYSICAL

Differentiating whether physical manifestations are caused by illness progression or exacerbation, infection or brought on as a response to emotional stress is very hard for ILD patients, their caregivers, and clinicians to determine. Therefore good, open dialogue is so essential in all discussions. It's easy for patients to get the impression that they are expected to be strong and find ways to cope while they might be feeling as if they are paddling just to stay afloat. Here is a non-exhaustive list of the many physical symptoms we experience when we are stressed:

- Low energy or fatigue
- Headaches
- Bruxing or jaw clenching
- Muscle cramps or tension chest pain
- Racing heartbeat

- Palpitations
- Generally shaky or nervous
- Cold hands and feet
- Gastric upsets
- Light-headedness or dizziness
- Upturned sleep pattern
- Frequent colds or infections
- Low sex drive or interest

Feeling in control is one of the most powerful things we can do for ourselves. As we get more and more anxious and SOB gets worse, the important thing is to feel that we are gaining control of what is happening. Just starting with breath control is worthwhile. Chapter 5 deals with this in greater detail but a brief description of breathing control here is still useful. Following are some tips on how to do that:

SLOWING THE BREATHING RATE

Start by slowing the rate of the breath; first breathing in for a count of 2 then out for 2, maintaining this for a few moments. Then continue in for 2 and out for 4 or whatever ratio you have found works for you. Combining this with pursed lip breathing is particularly useful when symptoms are increasing, and a sense of unease is developing fast.

PURSED LIP BREATHING

This is a type of breathing where we breathe in through the nose and exhale through the mouth gently. A visual could be smelling the roses and a very gentle blowing out through the mouth as if you are cooling soup. This can elicit more relaxed and easy breathing. With the relaxation that comes from feeling more in control of one's breath, other physical symptoms, such as racing pulse and palpitations are lessened. Go ahead – try it! It's important to reflect on how our emotions may be influencing our physical symptoms.

BEHAVIORAL

Sometimes we don't notice behavioral changes within ourselves, so it's worthwhile paying attention if someone else comments that our behavior is different from baseline. This can happen to any of us; patient, friend or caregiver and is so important to address, although it's not easy.

Below are some of the behavioral change's others might see that are brought on by stress. Remember that we are all different with different ways of behaving.

- Isolating socially
- Starting or refusing to consider stopping unhealthy habits.
- Putting off decisions of importance
- Developing nervous tics like pacing, nail biting
- Falling asleep in daytime but having difficulty at night

- Having outbursts of anger or irrational thoughts/ comments

COGNITIVE

Observing cognitive change brought on by stress is where we might start to get concerned about the emotional and mental well-being of ourselves or loved ones. When the signs below, often the result of negative self-talk and low self-esteem, are constant, it's time to act and seek professional support.

- Seeing only the negative in a situation.
- Unwanted thought or internal dialogue.
- Brain fog lacks concentration.
- Less discernment in judging or deciding.
- Acting anxious and finding it difficult to explain feelings or behavior.

All these behaviors throughout the grief stage of coming to terms with our diagnosis are perfectly understandable and normal. However, when they become more sustained, like a cloud enveloping us and our lives fall out of balance, that is when we need to pay more attention. Replacing negative self-talk with being more positive is a way forward. Like using the recovery breathing method to reduce the dreadful sensation of being SOB, try positive inner talk to get you through difficult times.

EMOTIONAL

Following are some of the more common emotional symptoms we might experience that are caused by anxiety, stress, and depression:

- Anxious thoughts, feelings, or behaviors
- Tense, mind turmoil causing difficulty sleeping.
- Depression or deep sadness
- Overwhelmed or feeling that thing are out of control
- Agitation, anger, irritability, or hostility
- Isolation from others and becoming lonely
- Less capable or low self esteem

Functions like breathing, heart rate and blood pressure are not usually what we spend much time thinking about until they stop operating automatically, which is controlled by the nervous system. Regulation of these functions come from a part of the nervous system called the autonomic nervous system which has three parts:

- The sympathetic system
- The parasympathetic system
- The enteric system

These work together by preparing us to face stressful situations, then return to a more relaxed state when it's over. This function is often described as the fight or flight response in a stressful scenario, but let's not forget that it also has day to day uses such as sweating to cool us down when the weather gets warm.

In fight or flight mode, the sympathetic system stimulates the release of adrenaline into the bloodstream. This increases our preparedness for action; our hearts might race; mouth feels dry and breathing becomes more intense. If we maintain that level of constant alert and having the body work overtime, we can cause serious health problems. In opposition, when the alert is over the parasympathetic will reduce our responses and allow the body to move into a rest and digest stage. Finding strategies to help us move out of the fight or flight stage is empowering and can bring calm and purpose to our lives.

The manifestations we have outlined can, if they become a regular occurrence, be a sign of a chronic stress situation. It can muddy the waters in situations where it mimics or exacerbates symptoms that come from having PF.

Now that we're aware of different stress responses and how they impact us physically, mentally, and emotionally, let's focus on countering the stress response.

EDUCATING OURSELVES

Learning more about this illness has been my (Grace) lifesaver. I admit that curiosity is a trait I have lived most of my life, but I also know that it has reduced my fear of the unknown, or worse, my fear of the dreaded. I learned that life with the prognosis of PF could be influenced by lifestyle, like all aspects of well-being. I could not change the course of my illness, but I could influence the kind of life I would lead while living with it.

Educating ourselves can build the confidence that allows us to be our best advocate. It can help create a positive state of emotional well-being that reduces fear and many of the physical symptoms caused by stress, fear, or anxiety. We feel a sense of control by knowing more, as they say: knowledge is power!

REACH OUT!

There is a lot of evidence that our emotional well-being is significantly improved by social contact and support. Previously, we have emphasized the importance of building a clinical team. Emotionally, we feel supported when our team is in regular communication, and we feel more like a person vs. a number to them.

SUPPORT GROUPS

Dealing with challenging emotions such as anxiety and depression is increasingly difficult alone. Talking with friends and family can be very useful and can be a feel-good factor for us. Feeling heard and supported from fellow patients and those who truly understand our experience, is just one of the benefits a support group provides.

There are various online support groups, among them the Pulmonary Wellness Foundation, that have platforms with excellent sources of information for patients and caregivers. Much of the information is from patients who understand what it feels like to be a person with an ILD and who are at various stages of their illness. On many support sites, funny anecdotes provide laughter, which they say is the best medicine.

LAUGHTER

It's a fact that laughter can lower stress levels, decrease anxiety, and reduce depression. It can relieve both physical and emotional tension in our bodies by reducing the level of stress hormones in the blood and stimulating the release of endorphins, relieving pain, and promoting healthy immune function.

Generating laughter comes in many forms; may be from watching cartoons, phoning a funny friend, or even turning that smile in the mirror into a grin which can become a laugh. It really doesn't matter what form it takes but it's worth fitting in ways to laugh throughout the day for the amazing benefits it brings to our mental health and well-being.

EATING WELL AND BEING NUTRITIONALLY WELL

While fighting a chronic illness, it's important to give our bodies as much good nutrition as possible by eating well, which is why we have devoted a chapter to nutrition in this book. Being emotionally healthy and committed to good nutrition influences what we eat, but what about the other way around? Large quantities of simple carbohydrates, sugars and refined foods are connected to negative emotions. This is not to say that a Belgian chocolate eclair is banned forever but keep it balanced.

Alcohol is a central nervous system depressant and while it may be enjoyable in the moment, it does have longer term negative consequences to our physical and emotional health. Additionally, caffeine drinks like tea, sodas and coffee can give a temporary stimulus and can also increase the negative feelings that are common in depression, anxiety, and stress.

PHYSICAL CONTACT

Physical contact or touch can be hard when you live on your own or have lost a partner, however, there are therapies like massage whose benefits go beyond the blissful relaxation that is so beneficial. Massage therapy can improve emotional health by increasing serotonin, a hormone that reduces depression and pain by enhancing the immune function. This also builds resistance to bacterial and viral illnesses.

PHYSICAL THERAPIES

There are a variety of physical therapies that can aid in relaxation. Massage is one of them, which may help us in unsuspecting ways. As my (Grace) PF has progressed, there has been a reduction in my ribcage depth. This has caused my posture to shift to a more forward head position, which causes the rib cage and lungs to be under even more physical pressure. When I have a massage, the muscles at the front of the ribcage relax and the back one's tone so I stand straighter. Emotionally, it feels better to be upright, facing the world, rather than curled up and feeling cowed. It also seems to expand my breathing ability no matter what the function tests show.

ROUTINE

Routine and consistency are an important aspect of mental health and well-being. This is especially true for those living with a chronic illness. It can be one less thing for us to think about and plan; allowing us to conserve both mental and physical energy. How we start our day can "set the scene" for good mental health. Personally, my (Grace) routine has changed from time to time while learning to cope with this illness.

Big changes, like developing pericarditis and atrial fibrillation, left me feeling despondent that I was deconditioned. That is where having the routine of Bootcamp, which is described in the exercise chapter, was crucial in emotionally helping me get back on my feet and re-establishing my daily routine. Linda also reminds us that establishing a routine may be as simple as identifying and committing to the completion of one small task. Or it could be a full day mapped out with precision.

Presently, I only concentrate on a few things. It includes a short gratitude meditation when I wake up, a smile in the mirror (after all who else is going to give me a smile today) and a qigong exercise to aid my breathing and develop energy. With these completed, the endorphins are kicking in and the day is already made better with this routine.

RELAXATION TECHNIQUES

There are a range of movement theories such as tai chi, yoga and qi gong that are associated with improved well-being and relaxation. The fluid movements that are part of these, together with breath control and mental focus, combine to produce a sense of calm. More restful bodily responses are achieved, and we feel more rested and less stressed. The mind-body connection is strong; one influences the other and finding a balance here reduces our pain and anxiety. Classes in these movement theories can be found in most communities and online. Participating in a class is a great way to obtain these benefits at any stage of your disease. Following are a few suggestions of how movements based on qigong can help, especially on those bad days when SOB is causing anxiety.

We sought the help of Brian Trzaskos, PT, LMT, CSCS, CMP, MI-C the creator of the Qigong for Pulmonary Health and founder and director of the Institute for Rehabilitative Qigong and Tai Chi (www.IROTC.com) who produced the following piece on universe tapping for breath anxiety. It is specifically for patients who are experiencing bad days; you know the ones when it all just seems like it's too much.

UNIVERSE TAPPING FOR BREATH ANXIETY by Brian Trzaskos

One of the most common issues associated with shortness of breath is that of anxiety. This makes perfect sense and is completely normal for anyone, with or without a pulmonary health condition, as fear of suffocation is one of only three primary fears that we are born with. Fortunately, there is a simple and effective tool for minimizing the anxiety that is associated with shortness of breath.

Like Qigong, Universe (aka Primordial) Tapping is a practice thousands of years old originating as a part of Traditional Chinese Medicine (TCM). TCM identifies 2,400 acupuncture points which act as "gateways" to energy channels or meridians in the body. TCM theory holds that when the body becomes chronically tense that energy or "qi" gets stuck in the meridians and is unable to circulate freely. Freely circulating "qi" is associated with good health and stuck or depleted "qi" is associated with disease. Tapping on certain acupuncture points has been shown to increase "qi" circulation, resulting in lower body tension, deeper breathing, decreased pain, less anxiety, and overall relaxation.

Going a bit deeper than the body responses to meridian tapping alone, TCM also teaches that our emotions have an energetic component as well. Emotions like fear, anger, grief, and anxiety can also become trapped in the body when "qi" is unable to circulate. To address this, Universe Tapping additionally includes a process of learning to accept what is happening in the moment while simultaneously releasing trapped emotions through positive affirmations.

Here are the steps to lowering your anxiety and breathing easier in just a few minutes:

Step 1: Using one or both hands, begin lightly tapping the following points for approximately 10-30 seconds each: the top of your head, over your eyebrows, the side of your eyes, under your eyes, under your nose, center of your chin, collarbones, under your arms, and sternum

Go through all the points, allow yourself to relax as you focus solely on the sensation of your fingers tapping the points. Very often this alone will help a person's breathing deepen; if so, just go with the flow and take some deeper breaths.

Step 2: Come up with a statement that includes both your primary concern and a positive vision of support from the Universe. Some examples would be:

- Even though I feel short of breath, I know calming myself will help me get through this episode."
- "Even though I feel short of breath, I have the tools to help myself."
- "Even though I feel short of breath, I release this anxiety to the Universe".

Feel free to modify your statement as you tap to allow it to feel supportive and relaxing. The secret to success is first to accept what is happening, followed by a statement of faith that despite how it may appear the Universe is loving and supportive. If you are a religious person, feel free to substitute your own loving God in the place of the Universe

Step 3: Continue lightly tapping the points and begin repeating your statement quietly internally or with a whisper. Cycle through tapping each point for 10-30 seconds while repeating your statement until you feel more settled and relaxed, allowing yourself to take a few deeper breaths.

These techniques are ways of harvesting energy, and we know how low that can be on occasions with PF. Brian's recommendation are to help reduce the emotional trauma that we encounter when we are dealing with SOB.

MEDITATION AND MINDFULNESS

Practicing meditation and mindfulness is widely known to be beneficial to counter negative emotions. There are countless apps and tools available to assist us with meditation. However, it can still feel daunting for some people, so it's worth remembering that any meditation practice allows us to slow down; reducing any physical or emotional responses that cause us problems. The very act of stopping and concentrating on a moment that is now can be an experience akin to meditation. As Rene says, "I have not formally practiced the art of meditation. Sharing a glass of wine while watching an amazing sunset and reminiscing over the wonderful places we have visited has a similar sensation for me".

Even with all these strategies in place, it's important to listen to ourselves if we are overwhelmed in a way that feels there is no way out. This may be the time when therapeutic counselling could be helpful. One aspect of the emotional turmoil that patients with a diagnosis of a chronic illness experience, could be compared to post traumatic stress disorder (PTSD). With PTSD symptoms, they are not a result of one single traumatic event, but one that is an ongoing threat to a person's sense of safety.

According to the National Centre for PTSD, this disorder can produce higher inflammatory levels in the body and subsequent behaviors such as having difficulty in adhering to medical treatment, avoiding, or messing up medications, or a patient's inability to follow up with appointments might occur. In an ideal world, it would be good if these behaviors raised alarm bells to clinicians that patients could be experiencing PTSD but that may not happen in a busy clinical environment. The extreme anxiety some of us feel at the time when diagnosis is given can be felt again on subsequent visits to the hospital. As a result, patients can find it difficult to assimilate information, leading to further potential for misunderstanding and lowered compliance.

When patients are experiencing PTSD, avoidance may seem like the only way out of a situation that is so deeply painful. This is a good reason to be seeking professional counselling. The intention behind counselling in this scenario is to help develop coping skills. A counselor or therapist can enable you to see the steppingstones to help deal with anxiety and depression which can deplete energy and prevent us from moving forward.

HOPE

Psychiatrist Victor Frankl wrote about his experiences with emotional health in 1959. More specifically, he talks about emotional health being influenced by the attitudes we choose, the decisions we make, and the desire to look forward rather than backwards. In the pursuit of optimal emotional well-being as we live with an ILD diagnosis, it's important to think about hope. While hope ebbs and flows throughout the course of our illness, it can be found in that space between despair and delusion.

In the negative state of despair, it feels like there is no way forward and the future holds no hope for improvement or happiness.

Delusion, on the other hand, can deny that there is no cure and placing faith in spurious activities. Hope reduces feelings of helplessness, increases happiness, reduces stress, and improves quality of life. It helps develop coping skills even though there is often confusion between hoping and coping.

In coping, we rely on processes or skills that help us deal with a particular situation, such as the use of controlled breathing for SOB. Good coping skills such as journaling, visualization, and meditation, can help us sustain hope; adjusting our approach when necessary, and allowing us to live our best lives.

If we consider that despite a diagnosis of PF, we can survive and cope with adversities, then we can heal and become accepting. This healing may not happen immediately, and it may not be physical, since a cure does not currently exist for PF. However, we are now in a better place to cope with the symptoms of PF and having a life-threatening lung disease. We can thrive when how we cope elicits hope for a life of positivity and emotional wellness.

Reference: https://www.ptsd.va.gov/publications/rq_docs/ V29N4.pdf

Chapter 15:

Prevention of Infection by Noah Greenspan, PT, DPT, CCS, EMT-B

"An ounce of prevention is worth a pound of cure." – Ben Franklin

Living with a chronic illness, particularly a respiratory condition can significantly compromise your immune system, making you more susceptible to picking up a bug, catching a cold or developing an infection or exacerbation of your existing pulmonary condition. Patients often report getting sick once, twice, three times or more over the course of a given year and whether it is a cold, the flu, pneumonia, or an exacerbation, it *always* seems to settle in the chest.

Frequent illnesses or exacerbations, or even one bad one, can impact the progression of your disease and its associated symptoms. For this reason, it is crucial not only to take care of yourself when you get sick, but also, that you take specific measures to PREVENT yourself from getting sick in the first place.

One thing that is important to realize is that even if you do everything right, you can *still* get sick anyway. However, our goals are to decrease the probability of your getting sick in the first place, increase your ability to fight off and recover from illness, and reduce the severity of that illness, when you do get sick, minimizing its impact on your life.

How We Get Sick

At the most basic level, disease is caused by pathogens. The most encountered pathogens are bacterial, viral, fungal, or parasitic in origin. The most common routes of transmission include airborne or inhaled, direct contact, indirect contact or contact with a contaminated surface, sexual contact, contact with infected blood or body fluids, and the fecal-oral route.

Viruses and bacteria cause most respiratory infections and unless you are living in a bubble, you will likely encounter one (or a million) of these daily. They are introduced to our bodies, through the mucus membranes of the eyes, nose, and mouth, either by inhaling them or by touching or coming into contact with a contaminated surface, and then touching your face.

We are also exposed to, and come into contact with spaces, surfaces and objects that are exposed to and contacted by many people daily. Anything that is touched by many people, many times each day has a greater chance of being contaminated with bacteria, viruses, and other pathogens.

Depending upon the type of organism and the surface on which they are found, some viruses and bacteria can live outside the body for up to 24 hours. Whether or not you get sick depends upon the specific virus or bacteria and the status of your own immune system.

Please understand that I am not trying to scare you into hermetically sealing yourself in bubble wrap. What I am trying to do is raise your awareness of everyday potential exposures so you can better protect yourself against them. Here are some suggestions on how to do that:

"Don't Patchke Your Face"

My Grandma Peppie used to say: "don't patchke your face." Patchke is a Yiddish word that means to play around or fiddle with. It was good advice then and it's good advice now. As I mentioned previously, pathogens are introduced to our bodies, through the mucus membranes of the eyes, nose, and mouth. So don't fiddle.

Wash your Hands (a lot)!

This goes hand in hand (pun intended) with "don't patchke your face." Frequent hand washing is your single best defense against introducing viruses or bacteria into your system. Most of us know (or should know) that we're supposed to wash our hands before we eat, or after we use the bathroom. However, that's not adequate, particularly for someone living with a pulmonary disease. You really need to be washing your hands every time you come in contact with a potential source of infection.

Also, to be clear, when we talk about hand washing that does not just mean a quick rinse. *Effective* hand washing means using soap and water, and rubbing your hands together *vigorously*, for at least 30 seconds. Keeping in mind that you initially turned the water *on* with dirty hands, turn it off using a paper towel so that you don't contact those germs again. The same goes for the bathroom door.

Antibacterial Gels/Creams/Lotions

If you don't have access to soap and water, carrying a small bottle of anti-bacterial gel, cream, or lotion can come in "handy". Some people may argue against using anti-bacterial products, on the grounds that they kill the good bacteria along with the bad. While this may be true to some degree, I would still choose using an anti-bacterial gel over walking around with the common cold or pneumonia or Covid on my hands, just waiting for an opportunity to enter my mucus membranes.

Antibacterial Sprays and Wipes

Remember also that objects or surfaces that you come in contact with may not be cleaned frequently (or ever), and therefore, may be contaminated with a whole host of pathogens. For this reason, it is well worth your time and effort to spray or wipe them with disinfectant before you use them. As just one example, when you go to the supermarket, wipe down the shopping cart before leaning all over it or putting your food inside.

At the Pulmonary Wellness & Rehabilitation Center, we have dispensers with anti-bacterial foam for our patients and staff. We also wipe down every machine in between every patient. The last thing we want is for people to get sick *at a wellness center*.

Protect Your Home

When you return home after a day out, you carry with you all of those nasty 'bugs' (bacteria and viruses) that have latched onto you and your belongings over the course of your day. You can help minimize their impact and reduce the likelihood of contaminating your home by taking a few precautionary measures.

First, as previously mentioned, wash your hands as soon as you walk in the door, and even better, take a shower. Change out of your dirty "outside clothes," and into your clean "inside clothes," and swap outside shoes for inside shoes or slippers.

When visitors enter your home, ask them to take similar precautions. Well, maybe not the shower part, but they can certainly take off their coats in the hallway, remove their shoes at the door, and wash their hands when they arrive. This is even more important when children are visiting. Since children are much more likely to come in contact with dirt, viruses, and bacteria, it would be to *everyone's* advantage if they have an extra set of clothes to change into and immediately wash up, especially after they've been playing outside.

Protect Your Property (O$_2$ Equipment and Supplies)

If you use oxygen, it is important to protect all your supplies and equipment including the tank or concentrator itself as well as all the accessories including tubing, masks, and cannulas. All the bugs that can travel with you on your clothes and your property, can also travel on your oxygen equipment. Be aware of where you place your equipment both at home and when you are out and wipe it down frequently with an antibacterial wipe, especially when returning home. With respect to your cannula or mask, be sure to place them on something clean when not in use and wipe them down if they have been sitting for a while. I can't tell you how many times, I have seen people's cannula hanging on the floor or thrown into their bag unprotected. If you keep it in a plastic bag, wipe it down BEFORE you put it in the bag and…wipe down the bag.

Be Aware of Your Surroundings

Equally important to being vigilant at home is minimizing your risk of exposure when you are out. As mentioned previously, this is particularly important when you are in public places that are regularly frequented by a lot of people.

Again, think about how many people's hands touch the handrails on escalators or stairs, equipment at the gym, door handles or push buttons. I'll give you a hint. It's *a lot*. And the poles on buses and subways are virtual petri dishes for every disease known to man and probably a few yet-undiscovered ones as well.

And then…there's the doctor's office. Now, that's a whole 'nother ball of bacteria (and viruses). Besides the obvious, *coming-in-contact-with-a-high concentration-of-sick-people-in-one-place*, how often do they clean the tables and chairs? And what about that annoying pen on a chain? Or even the magazines? If in doubt, don't be afraid to confirm that the area and equipment have been disinfected. While this may seem like an imposition on the staff, as healthcare professionals they should appreciate your concern and understand that it's better to be safe than sorry (or sick). As Ron Reagan said: "Trust but verify."

Dining Out

Dining out comes with its own unique risks of exposure to bacteria and viruses at every stage of the process, from the food preparation to its distribution, to its consumption. Every person, from the host or hostess to the chef, to the server, and every item from the table, to the menus, to the plates and utensils, to the food itself is a potential source of contamination. A weak link in any of these areas can increase your risk of exposure and illness. I don't know about you, but if I go into a restaurant and my server is sick, I simply excuse myself, leave a tip, and make it my business to get the heck out of there as fast as I can.

Other Factors

You can't make the whole world germ-free. However, you can do your best to protect yourself. Here are some other suggestions:

Stay Away from Sick People

That may sound overly simplistic, or even harsh in some cases, but it is both completely true and very important. Of course, we understand that you want to see your friends and family, but trust me, if your children are sick (or even your grandchildren), it is much better to take a rain check—for *everyone*. As someone with a chronic pulmonary disease, a cold for you is not the same as a cold for someone with a healthy immune system, and as heart-breaking as it might be to skip the visit; you really must look at the big picture. If that visit lands you in the hospital, it doesn't do anyone any good.

Stay at Home When You're Sick

Rule Number One: if you are sick, just stay home! We are condi-tioned to believe that we should never, ever, *ever* miss a day of work. However, that is a surefire way to prolong your illness and *maximize* its spread to as many people...and places...and surfaces as possible.

At the Center, our policy is if you are sick, you stay home, no if's, and's or but's. This applies to patients and staff alike, even if you feel well enough to exercise or come to work. Again, the last thing we want is for you to get sick at a wellness center or for you to get someone else sick at a wellness center (or anywhere else).

Get the Flu Shot

Many people ask whether they should get the flu shot. While there is no single best answer for everyone, the Center for Disease Control recommends that everyone 6 months or over should get the flu shot annually. This is especially true for people over 65, or anyone with a medical condition that could compromise their immune system such as respiratory and cardiovascular disease. However, individual cases will vary depending on age, level of risk, medical condition(s), and doctor preference, among other factors, so to be sure, check with your personal physician.

Get the Pneumonia Vaccine

Like the flu shot, there is no single best answer for everyone and again, individual situations will vary, so to be sure, please consult your personal physician. Up until recently, it was generally recommended that people over 65, or anyone with a medical condition that could compromise their immune system, get a one-time, single-dose vaccine, called the "pneumococcal polysaccharide vaccine 23 (PPSV23). However, based upon the findings of a large clinical trial, that recommendation has changed. At the time of this writing, the CDC recommendations are as follows:

- In addition to a single dose of PPSV23, at-risk individuals, 65 years of age or older, should also get a dose of the pneumo-coccal conjugate vaccine 13 (PCV13), which provides protection against community-acquired pneumococcal pneumonia and other *pneumonia* infections.
- People who have never had the pneumonia vaccine should get the PCV13 FIRST and get the PPSV23 six to twelve months later.
- People who have already had the PPSV23 should also have the PCV13 if it has been at least one year since their initial vaccination with PPSV23.

Get the Covid-19 Vaccine

At the time of this writing, most adults are on our first round of boosters for Covid-19 and children have begun getting their first doses. As a novel coronavirus that is still surging in many parts of the world, I am sure this situation will continue to evolve. Speak with your physician and continue to follow the latest guidelines from the CDC, NIH and WHO.

Get Enough Rest

Sleep affects every system of the body, from the immune to the endocrine, to the cardiovascular and pulmonary, and every other system in between, to some degree or another. Lack of sleep or not getting enough overall rest can have a negative impact on your body's immune system, lowering your body's resistance and its ability to defend itself against bacteria and viruses. While most guidelines recommend between 7 and 9 hours, the exact amount of sleep we need varies from individual to individual.

Don't Smoke!

Cigarette smoking is one of the worst possible things you can do to your body. As if causing heart disease, lung disease, cancer and complications during pregnancy weren't enough, smoking cigarettes also lowers your body's immune function and increases your chances of developing an infection or exacerbation. So just don't do it.

Avoid Triggers

In addition to bacteria, viruses and other pathogens that can make you sick, there are other substances and conditions that can act as "triggers." These triggers can cause a range of symptoms including irritation of the eyes, nose or throat, cough, tightness in the chest, shortness of breath, or inflammation of the airways and lungs. All these mechanisms of the inflammatory process can make you more susceptible to developing an illness or exacerbation.

Triggers can be more universal in scale like air pollution or weather, or they can be more personal and individualized like encountering a strong odor or cigarette smoke. Here are some of the more common triggers that can particularly affect people with respiratory disease:

Indoor Allergens

Indoor Allergens include things like dust, mold, cockroaches and roach droppings, and pets and animal dander, among others. Symptoms can include, coughing, sneezing, stuffy or runny nose, as well as itching, burning or tightness in the ears, eyes, nose, mouth, throat, or chest. In these situations, it is crucial to eliminate the source of exposure, whenever possible OR to remove yourself from the exposure. This can be difficult in each of the above situations, for various reasons. However, the longer time that you are exposed and the more intense the exposure, the greater the chances are and the greater the potential damage that you are likely to experience.

Outdoor Allergens

Outdoor Allergens include things like pollen, trees, grass, weeds, and mold, among others. Like indoor allergens, symptoms can include, coughing, sneezing, stuffy or runny nose, as well as itching, burning or tightness in the ears, eyes, nose, mouth, throat, or chest. These allergies will likely be greatest from the spring through the fall and your best bet is to avoid exposure as best you can. If you are exposed, treat it similarly to exposure to a virus or bacteria by washing your hands frequently and changing your clothes and showering when you come back home. Saline eyewashes may be beneficial as well as nasal and oral saline rinses. Pay attention to the local pollen and other allergen counts and speak with your doctor about any over the counter or prescription medications that might be helpful.

Pollution

People living in more industrialized, densely populated urban areas will likely be more exposed to pollution than those that live in areas that are more rural, sparsely populated and less industrial. Air pollution includes various gases, ozone in particular, smoke, haze, smog, and ash, among others. Depending upon where you live and the type of pollutants, the conditions can change seasonally, daily, or even over the course of a single day. In the case of environmental incidents or emergencies, conditions can change rapidly and dramatically.

Pollution will typically be worst on hot, humid days in the city. The Environmental Protection Agency (EPA) reports the Air Quality Index (AQI), which measures air quality based upon 5 pollutants: ground level ozone, particle pollution, carbon monoxide (CO), sulfur dioxide (SO2), and nitrogen dioxide (NO2). It is ground-level ozone and airborne particulate pollution that pose the greatest threat to humans (and animals), particularly, those in high-risk groups, like respiratory disease.

Check the AQI at www.airnow.gov if you plan on being outside for any significant period. On days when the air quality is poor (greater than 100), consider limiting your time outdoors and avoid strenuous activity. Since ozone is generally higher in the afternoon and evening, try to organize your day, accordingly, going out in the morning instead of later in the day.

Occupational Exposure

Certain jobs, hobbies and other activities will increase your chances of being exposed to one or more substances that can cause or worsen your respiratory condition. These include toxic chemicals and other irritants such as smoke, asbestos, dust, dirt, and debris, among many others. Ideally, you will be able to avoid this type of work but if this is not possible, be sure to be aware of and *use* maximum personal protection equipment (PPE) for the type and level of risk involved. This includes protective masks, gowns, gloves as well as any other specific protective gear for the task at hand.

Weather

Many people are affected by weather, particularly, either by heat and humidity or by cold, dry air. When it is hot and humid outside, the air seems to be thicker and heavier. As a result, people with respiratory disease are forced to work harder with each breath to move air in and out. When it is particularly hot and humid, try to go out early in the morning before the sun is at its strongest or in the late afternoon or evening, after the sun has begun to go down.

On cold, dry days, the airways can become narrower due to bronchoconstriction and spasm of the smooth muscle lining the airways. Ask your doctor if you can take your rescue inhaler or nebulizer about 15 minutes *before* going out. Also, cover your nose and mouth with a scarf, mask or other product that can help warm the incoming air.

Other Exposures

There are other exposures that are more personal, individual, or situational in nature and while I can't possibly name them all, here are a few examples:

- Cigarette (or other) smoke
- Perfumes, colognes and other scented oils or lotions
- Air fresheners, candles, and incense
- Construction

- Cleaning products
- Other

Again, I am not trying to scare the bejesus out of you. However, in many cases, depending upon the type, severity, and degree or intensity, one exposure can sometimes be enough to cause a problem, especially if you are already compromised in one way or another; to trigger inflammation or an exacerbation, or to get you sick. So, please take the extra time and effort to protect yourself and your loved ones.

Don't Shake Hands or Kiss Hello and Goodbye

While it may be customary to shake hands when you meet some-one, it is not in your best interest. Now, I'm not trying to be gross, but in most cases, you really have no idea when that person last washed their hands. In this situation, social mores must take a back seat to your health. The same goes for the hello and goodbye kiss and doubly so for the double kisses. You get the idea.

You can try using an alternative greeting: say "Namaste", bow, wave, or salute each other. Hell, throwing up a gang sign (joke). Or you can simply let people know that you don't shake hands. Whether or not you tell them the reason is up to you, but it could be a good teaching opportunity and a chance to educate others about your condition. The choice is yours. No pressure.

Throw Tissues Away Immediately After Use

This one may seem obvious, but I can't tell you how many people I see blowing their nose and then putting the dirty tissue back in their pocket, purse, up their sleeve, or in their bra (or what I like to call: "Grandma's tissue box") …and don't even get me started on the handkerchief! I don't know who thought of this brilliant idea, but do you really want to save that stuff for later? Besides being a treasure trove of bacteria, they're just gross. So don't use one.

Avoid Confined Spaces

Whenever possible, avoid spending prolonged periods of time in small, enclosed spaces with poor ventilation. Try to stay in large, open, well-ventilated areas with lots of fresh air and where close contact with others is less intense.

As an example, airplanes are one of the worst possible places when it comes to the transmission of illnesses for a whole host of reasons. There are lots of people, in close proximity to each other. The air is re-circulated around the cabin and the surfaces are rarely disinfected. This makes it very easy for bacteria or viruses to travel from person to person, on surfaces or through the air. Although not quite as bad, the situation is similar in small offices, elevators, or other enclosed areas.

Suit Up

Let's face it. Regardless of how well we attempt to prepare ourselves for every possible condition, we are all going to encounter situations in which we have no control over our environment. When all else fails and you find that you cannot control the environment or those around you, more extreme measures must be taken. Suit up. When we know we are going to be in a hostile environment, wearing a mask and/or gloves can be an effective last-ditch effort to avoid exposure.

Seek Medical Attention Sooner Rather Than Later

By now, you should realize that I believe in the "better safe than sorry", "err on the side of caution," and "an ounce of prevention…" schools of thought. When in doubt, seek medical attention *sooner rather than later*. As I have mentioned on many occasions, a cold is not the same for me as it is for you or someone with a respiratory disease; and a day or two, and sometimes even a few hours, can be the difference between preventing and minimizing the impact of a problem versus really getting in trouble. Many doctors will give their patients a prescription for antibiotics and/or steroids to keep on hand for when they do get sick.

Other Suggestions

Recently, I asked the members of my Ultimate Pulmonary Wellness Facebook group to share some of their own personal practices for preventing infection. Here are some of their suggestions:

- Use antioxidant vitamins, minerals, and herbs; particularly, vitamin C, zinc, Echinacea, and green teas
- Use immune-boosting products like "Airborne," "Emergen-C," or NUUN.
- Use gut health-enhancing probiotics
- Use nasal rinses and throat gargles
- Use an air filter/purifier

Chapter 16:

Airway Clearance by Marion Mackles, BS, PT, LMT and Noah Greenspan

"Out, damned spot! out, I say!" – Lady Macbeth

Everyone has mucus. It is one of the many defense mechanisms in our body's arsenal that protect us against infection and other *un*-pleasantries. In fact, if Lady Macbeth were a chest physiotherapist, she may well have been known for another quote: "Out, damned snot!" Before we discuss how to minimize and mobilize the secretions (mucus) that may accumulate in your airways because of your disease, it will be helpful for you to have a basic knowledge of what mucus is and what mucus actually does.

Take a breath in through your nose. Congratulations! You have just inhaled a small sample of the many thousands of tiny organisms and a varied array of particulate matter that we breathe in each day. When we breathe in through the nose, the air goes through its first warming, filtering, and humidifying process. If you are a mouth breather, the respiratory tissues will have to handle the job on their own, further down the respiratory tract.

The mucous (different than mucus) tissues or *membranes* that line the nasal cavity have a sticky surface that helps trap debris, like flypaper. There are also tiny hair-like structures called *cilia that* help move the air and mucus through the sinus cavity to prepare it for its journey into the lungs, the GI tract; or to be expectorated.

Our airways and lungs perform a similar filtration process as air passes through them. This filtration system is called the *"mucociliary escalator,"* or *"mucociliary transport system."*

The Airway Swamp

The airways leading into the lungs are lined with epithelial cells that protect the airways and lungs. These cells are loosely square-shaped and have thousands of cilia. Scattered throughout the epithelial cells are mucus-producing goblet cells. This is where I start to draw a picture in my mind of a swamp. The cilia float in a thin mucous fluid that is slightly thicker than water and a thick layer of mucus that rests on top of the cilia. That's the stuff that traps debris; which I like to picture as bugs in the swamp; that are stuck to the top scummy layer.

Under all of that, we have clear, crisp water in which our cilia (swamp plants) move back and forth in a wave-like motion. This wave-like motion pushes the mucus up through the airways, millimeter by millimeter to the throat, where it is either swallowed or expectorated (coughed out). If it is swallowed, the stomach acids destroy any organisms that may be living in the mucus. In addition, to swallowing or expectorating, some smaller particles of mucus are expelled as vapor when we exhale. This process automatically takes place every second of every day, whether we have a pulmonary condition or not.

Just like the ecosystem of a swamp, any alien intruder or other irritant can throw this well-coordinated system out of balance. In response, the goblet cells start *overproducing* mucus to help fight whatever irritant or foreign invader may be present. In addition, goblet cells from the lower layers can break through to the upper layer, overpowering the ciliated epithelial cells. At this point, we lose the wave action of the cilia, and the sluggish goblet cells take over the swamp. This delicate transport system can also be affected by other factors like scar tissue or paralyzed cilia (from cigarette smoking or exposure to environmental toxins), temperature, and humidity.

AIRWAY CLEARANCE TECHNIQUES

When it comes to airway clearance techniques, patients often ask, "which method works the best?" and the answer is always the same: "it depends on the individual." Every person is *at least* slightly different with respect to his or her anatomy and physiology, disease process and progression, level of conditioning, lifestyle, etcetera, and etcetera. For that reason, it will often take some trial and error to figure out what will work best *for you*, but at some point, you must take the first step. Starting somewhere and doing *something* is always better than doing nothing!

When it comes to the techniques themselves, you have many options available to you, including the many devices on the market such as positive expiratory pressure (PEP) devices, oscillating PEP devices, valves that alter sound wave frequencies, and vests, among others. There are also manual chest therapy techniques that require a second person to assist you. However, before we get to those, let's talk about some of the techniques you can do on your own and without spending a penny. These techniques can be used on their own *or* in tandem with one of the various devices to make the treatment even more effective.

I usually recommend performing the airway clearance techniques two to three times per day. The most important (and effective) times are in the morning, shortly after you wake up and in the evening about an hour or so before going to bed, *not* immediately before bed. Sometimes, it can take a while for the mucus to come up and we don't want your sleep to be disturbed by coughing. Many of the positions people sleep in are also natural drainage positions (which we will discuss later). Did you ever notice that when you wake up in the morning, one of the first things you do is clear your throat, cough, or even hack up some sputum? This is the perfect time to take advantage of Mother Nature by using one of the clearance techniques for maximum benefit.

In the evening, you want to clear out your lungs of whatever may have accumulated during the day. These times can also be coordinated with your medications. Some techniques work well 5–15 minutes after taking your bronchodilator. Vests and some of the other devices can be used *while* nebulizing to help the medications go deeper into the lungs. But, before we get too far ahead of ourselves, let's look at the techniques.

Active Cycle of Breathing Technique (ACBT)

The *Active Cycle of Breathing (ACBT)* consists of a series of different breathing patterns that help loosen and mobilize mucus for expectoration, i.e., huffing, coughing, or in some cases, "hacking out" the mucus. ACBT requires no equipment and can either be performed sitting in a chair or in one of the postural drainage positions. For most sessions, I prefer not to have patients leaning back in the chair. When you lean back and rest on a surface, you are inhibiting ribcage movement and airflow to that part of the lungs. Instead, sit straight up with your feet flat on the floor. Please check with your physician before trying these techniques and if possible, schedule a session with a chest physical therapist or health professional trained in ACBT. If this is not possible, begin your practice slowly with the basic cycle.

A. Breathing Control or Relaxed Breathing (1 minute)

Settle into a relaxed, gentle, pattern of breathing in through the nose and exhaling quietly (not forced) through pursed lips, although some people teach this with an open mouth. If you have difficulty breathing in through your nose, breathe in through pursed lips. This step will relax the airways and accessory muscles and can also help alleviate anxiety. Breathing control should always be done before a huff (more on this in a moment).

B. Deep Breathing or Thoracic Expansion (3–5 breaths)

While taking a slow, deep, breath in, expand your lower ribs, allowing air to fill your chest. Don't force it! You may want to do this in front of a mirror placing your hands on your lower ribs when you are first learning this technique. Once your lungs are full, hold your breath for 2–3 seconds. If you are uncomfortable with breath holding (or prone to pneumothorax), you can skip this step. Then, sigh your breath out through pursed lips, allowing your ribcage to deflate slowly, like an accordion.

C. Huffing or Forced Exhalation (1–3 breaths)

Huffs are a form of forced exhalation. To do this, open your mouth wide with a relaxed dropped jaw. Imagine that you are trying to steam up your glasses before you clean them.

The basic pattern is ABAC, which equals one cycle:

A. Breathing Control or Relaxed Breathing (1 minute)
B. Deep Breathing or Thoracic Expansion (3–5 breaths)
A. Breathing Control or Relaxed Breathing (1 minute)
C. Huffing or Forced Exhalation (1–3 breaths)

I recommend repeating the cycle until you have expectorated, but no more than 3 times so you don't wear yourself out. Often, a patient will become very productive about a half hour to an hour *after* ACBT.

There are two different types of huffs:

C1: Lower Airway Huff:

Take a small to medium breath in and give an extended huff out. The lower airway huff clears secretions from your lower airways.

C2: Upper Airway Huff:

Take a long, slow, deep breath in and give a quick huff out. The upper airway huff clears secretions from your upper airways.

If you choose to do both types of huffing, separate them by 1 minute of **Breathing Control** in between. Depending on your ability, or what works best for you, the cycle can be extended (e.g., ABABAC1). You can also perform several cycles (e.g., ABAC1/ABAC2/ABAC1). In this case, the pattern would be:

Cycle 1:

A. Breathing Control or Relaxed Breathing (1 minute)
B. Deep Breathing or Thoracic Expansion (3–5 breaths)
A. Breathing Control or Relaxed Breathing (1 minute)
C1. Lower Airway Huff (1–3 breaths)

Cycle 2:

A. Breathing Control or Relaxed Breathing (1 minute)
B. Deep Breathing or Thoracic Expansion (3–5 breaths)
A. Breathing Control or Relaxed Breathing (1 minute)
C2. Upper Airway Huff (1–3 breaths)

Cycle 3:

A. Breathing Control or Relaxed Breathing (1 minute)
B. Deep Breathing or Thoracic Expansion (3–5 breaths)
A. Breathing Control or Relaxed Breathing (1 minute)
C1. Lower Airway Huff (1–3 breaths)

There may be slight variations in the methods and techniques used, depending upon the physical therapist. However, as always, the individual protocols should be adapted to match the needs and abilities of the patient.

Controlled Cough

I like my patients to complete every chest clearance session with a 3-tier controlled cough. We are not talking about hard, forceful coughs that tighten the throat and irritate the tissues. When done properly, coughing is one of the most effective clearance tools.

Sit with your feet flat on the floor, shoulder-width apart. Place both hands on your abdomen, pressing slightly inward like a girdle. Take a slow, deep breath in through your nose and hold for 2–3 seconds. Then, bending forward, simultaneously give 3 small, short, staccato-type coughs in a single breath while continuing to apply pressure to your abdomen. If you need to repeat this process, perform 1 minute of breathing control/relaxed breathing before continuing.

Splinted Cough

If you need more support, you can wrap your arms around your abdomen or hug a pillow or towel. This is particularly helpful following thoracic or abdominal surgery. If this is the case, place the pillow or towel over the incision site and squeeze for added support and to reduce pain. This is also effective for anyone who might have musculoskeletal or orthopedic issues or osteoporosis that might be prone to spontaneous rib fractures, including people who have been on steroids for prolonged periods or at a high dosage.

Postural Drainage

Postural drainage consists of 12 different positions that use gravity to help mucus drain from the various lung segments into the larger airways, where it can be expectorated. I recommend holding each position for 5–15 minutes; and some specialists recommend even longer. Like everything else, you just must try it and learn what works best for you. Some people need to incorporate all the positions into their daily routine, while others only need to use one or two regularly.

Many patients benefit from leaning over a table while sitting or standing, performing deep breathing exercises. Some hang over their beds; or use a tub chair or bench. Sitting in the shower, they lean forward while splinting their arms on their legs or on the wall in front of them, while doing deep breathing or ACBT. Many people find that the steam from the shower helps loosen their secretions, making it easier for them to expectorate.

Postural drainage techniques are best done with ACBT. Many patients also use PEP devices to loosen the mucus even more while in these positions. Some people benefit from taking their bronchodilator 5–15 minutes *before* postural drainage and any nebulized steroids or antibiotics about 30 minutes to an hour *after* postural drainage.

NOTE: Do not eat for an hour before your postural drainage treatment.

In addition to the drainage positions alone, healthcare professionals can also use percussion (or cupping), vibration, and shaking when performing chest therapy and teach these techniques to family members or caregivers. In some positions, the patient can percuss himself/herself or use a small handheld vibrator. You can also buy handheld cupping devices that are specifically designed for chest therapy (not musculoskeletal treatments). As always, please find a trained health care professional to teach you and your caregivers the proper techniques and adaptations to suit your situation.

Percussion (Cupping)

Contrary to what some of you may have experienced, percussion or cupping does not involve hitting or slapping the stuffing out of somebody with an open hand. *When done properly*, this technique should *not* be painful at all. To perform cupping, gently cup your hand, clapping the chest wall in a rhythmic pattern, alternating hands. Instead of a slap, you should hear a hollow, popping sound and feel the flow of air passing between your hands. To protect the skin, the patient should wear a thin layer of clothing like a t-shirt or hospital gown. Keep in mind that you are *not* trying to bang the mucus out. What you *are* doing is vibrating air molecules to shake the mucus loose.

Vibration

Vibration involves placing a flat hand firmly over the focal area, typically over the ribcage. Keeping your own trunk stable, stiffen your arm and hand, causing it to shake. The patient should take deep breaths in through the nose and out through the mouth, with vibration being performed during exhalation. This technique along with cupping is extremely effective in helping to mobilize secretions.

Always end your sessions with some good deep breaths and controlled coughing (or huffs, or both). Again, please check with your doctor before beginning any chest therapy program, especially if you have any musculoskeletal or orthopedic issues, cardiovascular conditions, GERD (acid reflux/acid stomach), or hemoptysis (blood in your sputum).

Now that we have covered treatments you can do at home, mostly without help, and without purchasing anything, let's move on to the world of valves and other gizmos aka airway clearance devices.

Airway Clearance Devices

Incentive Spirometer (IS)

Many people ask about the incentive spirometer and may even have one hanging around from a previous hospital stay, particularly, following a thoracic, abdominal, or other surgical procedure. These plastic devices use plastic balls or a plunger-type indicator to provide a patient with visual feedback for inhaled airflow and volume. Using this device can help prevent atelectasis, pneumonia, and other pulmonary complications caused by prolonged bedrest, anesthesia, and/or pain medications. An incentive spirometer helps to clear secretions by visually cueing a person to take in a greater volume of air, opening the lungs more fully.

Some of our patients find that using an incentive spirometer helps them to take a few deeper breaths either prior to postural drainage or at the end, before performing a controlled cough. Anything that helps you take a deeper breath or mobilize secretions is a good thing!

The incentive spirometer comes with a list of settings of normal volumes based on age and gender. Start with a setting that is just *slightly* above the highest amount that you can currently perform, gradually increasing the volume as your lungs improve. We instruct our patients to take a slow, deep breath in through the nose and gently blow out through pursed lips. Then put the mouthpiece in your mouth with a tight seal and slowly inhale. When you get to your peak, hold the breath for 1–3 seconds and then let the air out gently. Some clinicians will ask you to blow the air out into the apparatus. I ask my patients to take the mouthpiece out and exhale through pursed lips.

Usually, people are instructed to repeat the process 10 times in a single sitting, but patients often start to fatigue their diaphragm, making this an exercise in futility. Instead, repeating only 3 cycles at a time, allows you to focus on the process, slowing things down and making it more effective, without becoming exhausted. The first time allows you to get a feel for the exercise, the second lets you make any necessary adaptations, and the third time is for the win! However, do not stress too much about performing an exact number of breaths or exhaling with or without the mouthpiece. Instead, try to focus on properly executing the *inhalation* through the mouthpiece. Always end your sessions with some deep breathing and controlled coughing (or huffs, or both).

POSITIVE EXPIRATORY PRESSURE VALVE

The PEP (Positive Expiratory Pressure) valve is not used as often but has been around since the 1970s. Once the oscillatory PEP valves (Flutter, Acapella) became available in the 1990s, many doctors, therapists, and patients switched over. On a PEP valve, you take a deep, full breath and exhale slowly through the mouthpiece. When blowing out, the device's resistance pressure (between 10–20 cm H2O) helps splint open the airways. This allows more air to move along the airways below the mucus to move it into the larger bronchi. Most of these devices have a manometer to ensure you are creating the right amount of pressure.

Once again, start in a comfortable seated position. Using your ACBT, perform 1 minute of breathing control relaxed breathing. This time, replace the deep breathing portion with 10 inhalations and exhalations through the PEP. Continue to follow your ACBT while substituting the deep breathing portion with the PEP device. To visualize this method, I like to think about the air flowing down the sides of airways, speeding by trapped cloud-like shapes of mucus. Then, I picture the air reaching a bulb-shaped bottom where it whips around for a high-speed return trip up the center of the airways, pushing the mucus up with it. Please note that as with all the PEP devices, make sure that you are not puffing your cheeks, which will diminish the effects. If you find that you do tend to puff your cheeks, use one hand to hold them while exhaling.

While positive expiratory pressure makes mucus clearance easier by opening the airways, it does not do anything to thin out or break up that hard-to-clear mucus—which brings us to oscillating PEP devices. In addition to providing positive expiratory pressure, these devices vibrate as you blow out.

Flutter Valve

The **Flutter Valve** made its US debut in late 1994 or early 1995 and is shaped like a small pipe. Inside, are a small cone-shaped funnel and a metal ball. As you blow out of the device, the ball bounces up and down, causing short spurts of intermittent positive expiratory pressure and a vibration that resonates and is amplified in the airways. The great thing about the **Flutter** is that it is small, durable, and easy to clean. However, the Flutter's success is highly dependent on proper positioning. You must be in an upright position (preferably sitting in a chair or sitting up in bed) with your chin slightly tilted upward. The device itself must be held at a certain angle with the stem (mouthpiece) parallel to the floor at approximately 15 degrees above or below parallel.

Many of our patients have trouble consistently finding the position that works best for them or achieving a vibration. However, when this device is used properly, it works well. Generally, once you have found a position where you feel a good resonant vibration in your upper airway and hear a good flutter sound from the pipe, sit in straight position with your feet flat on the floor and head tilted up (you can rest your elbows on a table to splint open the ribcage if you need). You are ready to begin the session.

The Flutter is used in 2 stages:

Stage 1: Mucus Loosening and Mobilization

Making sure that your lips have a tight seal on the mouthpiece, take a deep breath in to fill your lungs fully (but do not force the air in). Hold your breath for 2–3 seconds, and then blow out quickly but not forcefully. Your exhalation should be controlled and longer in duration than your inhalation. Remember; do not puff your cheeks. Repeat this step 5–10 times. I often ask my patients to perform 1 minute of relaxed breathing control before repeating another 5–10 breaths through the Flutter. During the first stage, it is important to try to suppress your coughs.

Stage 2: Mucus Elimination

Inhale deeply (totally filling your lungs). Hold this breath for 2–3 seconds, and then blow out as forcefully as possible. Try to empty your lungs completely. Repeat this cycle 1 more time followed by a cough (or a huff and a cough).

It takes a while to get a feel for the apparatus and to figure out how many breaths to do in Stage 1. Be patient with yourself.

The Acapella Vibratory PEP

A few years after the Flutter valve hit the market, the **Acapella Vibratory PEP System** showed up. The original **Acapella Blue DM** (a low-flow valve [<15L/min]) and **Acapella Green DH** (a high-flow valve [>15L/min]) are easier to use than the **Flutter**. The device consists of a body surrounding the inner works and a removable mouthpiece. The original device cannot be opened for proper cleaning and drying. Now, these original Acapella Green and Blue are marketed as single-use devices for use during an acute hospital or nursing care stay. The company now makes the **Acapella Choice** and **Acapella Duet**. Both open and can be taken apart for proper washing.

Both device versions have resistance dials to control the frequency of the vibration and the user does not have to be in any specific position for the apparatus to work. Therefore, you can use these devices in any of the drainage positions to increase their effectiveness. The Acapella Duet has a special port for a nebulizer system and a separate chamber for the nebulized medication, which wastes less medication. This device is sturdy and can be used with or without a nebulizer.

NOTE: All Acapella products can be attached to a nebulizer. Some attach directly, and some require an adapter to attach to the end of the device. When you nebulize with the Acapella, vibrations and PEP push the meds further into your airways. We often instruct our patients to wait 5 minutes after nebulizing with the Acapella, breathe in and out through the device about 3–5 times, and then cough.

After a quick search online, you will see there are as many ways to use the Acapella as there are days in the week. I find this device effective to use with **ACBT**, but I recommend switching it up so that you begin with the **deep breathing** portion. In other words, breathe in and out, slowly but strongly, through the device for 1 minute (10–15 breaths). Then, follow with **controlled, relaxed breathing** for 1 minute. Perform each step 3 times before coughing.

1. Start **deep breathing** in and out of the **Acapella** for 1 minute or 10–15 breaths—whichever comes first.
2. Switch to relaxed **breathing control** without the device in your mouth for 1 minute
3. Immediately put the Acapella back in your mouth for another round of **deep breathing** (1 minute) and **breathing control** (1 minute), followed by another round of **deep breathing** (1 minute), and **breathing control** (1 minute), for a total of 3 cycles.
4. Take a deep breath in, hold it for 2–3 seconds, and cough (or huff and cough—whatever works for you).

As with the **Flutter,** make a tight seal on the mouthpiece with your lips and keep your cheeks from puffing out. If possible, suppress your cough until the end of the third set of your relaxed breathing/ **breathing control**. If you need to cough badly, try to wait until you complete your set of **deep breathing** with the Acapella device.

There is one note to make about positioning of the device. The device must always be perpendicular to your nose (when sitting parallel to the floor), or it will not work well. If you maintain a 90-degree angle from your face with the device, it will work in any position that you place your body. For example, if your left side is totally congested, you can lay on your right side to inhibit air from going into that side and use the Acapella to focus your drainage on the left side.

The device does not work as well when it is moist. As a result, make sure you do not put the device back together after cleaning until it is thoroughly dry. Some people buy one device for the morning and one for the night so that they always have a clean, dry instrument.

THE AEROBIKA OSCILLATING PEP DEVICE

The **Aerobika Oscillating PEP (OPEP)** device is an incredibly convenient device that actually won an award for its design. It is very portable and lightweight. It comes apart easily for cleaning and can be put back together just as easily. Like the **Acapella**, it is not position-dependent and has a resistance setting.

Like the **Flutter** and **Acapella,** the **Aerobika** uses positive expiratory pressure to splint open the airways, while oscillations thin mucus and stimulate the cilia to mobilize secretions into the upper airways where they can be expectorated.

As with all these devices, make sure you have a tight seal on the mouthpiece, hold your breath for 2–3 seconds before you exhale into the device (we call it the "and" beat), make your exhalation 3–4 times greater than your inhalation, and keep your cheeks as stiff as possible (no puffing them out!). Again, if you find you are puffing your cheeks, use whichever hand is not holding the device to squeeze your cheeks. A manometer accessory can attach to the mouthpiece so that you have a visual gauge to determine whether you are achieving the right amount of pressure as you breathe out. The instructions for daily use from the company are also easy to follow. The manufacturer suggests breathing in and out through the apparatus for 10–20 breaths followed by 2–3 "huff coughs;" repeat this pattern for 10–20 minutes until you clear.

We use the same protocol for the **Aerobika** as we do for the **Acapella**. Once again, we use the **ACBT** switched up, starting with the **deep breathing** portion so that you start with 1 minute of breathing in slowly, but strongly, through the device (for approximately 10–15 breaths), followed by relaxed **breathing control** for 1 minute. Perform each step 3 times and then cough.

The **Aerobika** can also be used with a nebulizer. Many of our patients use this device with the nebulizing system that they already own. Monaghan, the maker of the **Aerobika,** also has their own nebulizer system (the **Aeroeclipse**), which has gotten great feedback from many of our patients. Again, if you are using the device while nebulizing, I often instruct our patients to wait 5 minutes after nebulizing with the Aerobika, and then breathe in and out through the device again (about 3–5 times), and cough.

If you use these devices for nebulizing, make sure you clean them well to prevent the medication from leaving a residue. Many of our patients will buy 2 of the same models and dedicate a device for nebulizing at home and the other for clearance without nebulizing that they carry around all day. Check with your doctor or health care professional before nebulizing with any device.

As an example, you may want to nebulize with a bronchodilator or saline solution, while using the device to open your airways or thin your mucus, respectively. Once you have cleared, nebulize with your other drugs without using the device. However, if you nebulize with medications such as anti-inflammatories or antibiotics, first clear with the device and nebulize without it. This is why it's so important to speak to and train with the proper healthcare providers. It also underscores the importance of knowing the medications you are taking—what they do and why you are taking them.

OTHER CLEARANCE DEVICES

Some patients and/or doctors occasionally ask about the **Lung Flute**, which is not actually a PEP device. It works via a low-frequency acoustical waveform produced when air is blown through the mouthpiece and over a long reed inside the device. This low-frequency wave travels to the lower airways and changes the viscosity of the mucus (making it thinner). The Flute's larger size makes it harder to carry around. It is easy to clean and comes with several months' worth of reeds. However, it can be difficult for people with weak hands or joint pain to change the reeds.

To use it, take a breath in before quickly and firmly inserting the mouthpiece and blowing into the Flute (as if you are gently blowing out a candle) for 20 sets of 2 breaths. You will hear the reed vibrate, but you will not feel a vibration like with the other devices. After each set of 2 breaths, rest for 5–10 seconds. When you are done, wait 5 minutes while secretions collect in the back of your throat. Then, cough for several minutes to bring up the secretions. The entire session usually takes about 5–10 minutes. Secretions may continue to collect for several hours after using the device.

Only a few of our patients use the **Lung Flute** because they complain that it fatigues them too much. Those who do best with this device are usually our younger and fitter asthma patients. Many patients will also use another device to clear after the 5-minute rest, prior to coughing. Some use the Flute in the morning to move the deeper secretions and use the Aerobika, Acapella, or another valve for their afternoon and/or night session.

There are a few other devices on the market that we do not see much in our practice, but occasionally a patient presents who uses one of them already or asks about it.

Another device is the **Quake**. It is small like the **Flutter** and is not position dependent. It cannot be used with a nebulizer. The **Quake** does have a very strong vibration on both inhalation and exhalation. However, patients struggle with the "handle" that controls the frequency of the vibrations that must be continuously manually rotated throughout the breathing part of the protocol.

For patients who can manage it, the **Quake** works well as a supplement for those who use other clearance devices but have difficulty bringing secretions up past their throat.

After using their other clearance device and coughing, they perform a minute of **breath control/relaxed breathing** followed by about 3–5 breaths in and out slowly through the **Quake** followed by another cough or huff. Reports from these patients have been positive.

This device has also helped some patients who aspirate food while swallowing. If they have the coordination and ability, I ask them to wait about 45 minutes after eating and then perform about 5 breaths in and out of the device, followed by a cough or huff. Often, they will cough up thin secretions with tiny food particles in them.

The **RC-Cornet/Curaplex VibraPEP** is another positive expiratory oscillatory device that is not position dependent, has an adjustable resistance valve, can be used with a nebulizer, and is reportedly easy to clean. It has a long, curved shape with a mouthpiece and a soft, flexible tube inside that vibrates on exhalation. I have never tried it, but word on the street is that it gets a "thumbs up."

Some patients benefit from high-frequency chest wall oscillation devices (**HFCWO**), also known as "vests." These devices involve wearing a vest or a wide wrap over the ribcage. They attach to tubes that are linked to a motor (generator). The vests fill with air, applying positive pressure to the outside of the ribcage. At the same time, the device pulses and shakes, causing air in the airways to vibrate, thinning and loosening secretions, and increasing airflow to move the mucus to the upper airways to be coughed out.

Some of our patients swear by these devices, but others hate them. Some disliked the brand they were using and eventually tried another, which they either loved or hated. **HFCWO**'s are big, heavy, and loud, making people less compliant when it comes to using them. Here's the rub: when they work for a patient, they work very well! You also can nebulize at the same time to get the medication deeper into the airways. I ask my patients who use these devices to perform relaxed breathing for a few minutes after completing their "vest" treatment, followed by 5–10 blows on a vibratory/oscillating PEP device to remove their secretions from the upper airways.

A portable **HFCWO** showed up in the US marketplace about 3 years ago, which has a portable battery and handheld remote. This allows you to be mobile while receiving your treatments. Patients often switch things up to make these tools work for them. Some people will pause their **HFCWO** machine every 5 minutes and use their PEP devices for 5–10 blows. Some nebulize for part of their session and stop it every 5 minutes to huff or take some blows on their PEP devices for the duration of their session.

Other tools are now on the market such as the *VibraLung* Acoustical Percussor Electro-Mechanical Acoustical Airway Clearance. The manufacturer's 40-plus-page booklet explains how it works much better than I can. Basically, instead of working on a single frequency like the other vibratory/oscillating PEP devices, it works on multiple frequencies at the same time.

The shorter the *wavelength*, the *higher* the frequency, and the *higher* the *pitch; higher pitches travel well in narrower airways, just like in the pipes of an organ. The opposite is true for wider airways.* While none of our patients use this device, the VibraLung may be worth looking into for people who might require a **HFCWO** but are unable to tolerate the pressure on their ribcage.

PUTTING YOUR DEVICE TO GOOD USE

At this point, I want to take a moment to talk about expectations. I always tell our patients that I see 4 types of results with these devices. The first type of patient is so productive that within a minute of starting to use the device, he or she starts to expectorate mucus.

The second type of person uses the device but does not produce any mucus until about 20 minutes to an hour later, at which point he or she becomes extremely productive and able to clear; some patients must take a few extra blows on their device at that time to make sure they have totally cleared.

A third group reports that nothing happens with the device, except that they feel less symptomatic and can breathe better (e.g., coughing less at night). I instruct this type of patient to continue to use the device until his or her next x-ray and/or CAT scan. Many times, the tests will also show some improvement. I am not sure why this happens, but my professional opinion is that the device is breaking up this patient's mucus enough for him or her to get rid of it naturally.

Finally, the fourth group reports no changes in their condition. In these cases, I check with their pulmonologists to make sure there are no new occurrences in the patient's disease processes. If everything comes back negative, we look at other techniques, protocols, and devices to use either separately or together.

Other great ways to clear are using the Pulmonica (a harmonica designed for pulmonary patients), singing (a fast-paced song works well), laughing, and exercise. Anything that forces you to take deeper breaths in and longer breaths out can reduce your mucus.

SUPPLEMENTING WITH THE "P-*HUH*" METHOD

One of my favorite techniques that our patients love is the "P-*huh*" technique. This is hard to explain on paper but let us give it a try. Tighten your lips like you are preparing to pop your "P." Take a deep breath in through your nose and hold it for a second or so. Next, push the air out of your mouth as if you want to throw it across a room, popping or emphasizing the "P" sound while saying "P-*huh*." It sort of sounds like a huff cough with an explosive "P" at the beginning. Once you master the initial "P-*huh*," you can move on to the exercise routine.

To do this, perform 3 sets of continuous "P-huh" sounds quickly and softly—as if you were reciting Shakespeare or a song from Hamilton:

1. Take a deep breath in and do as many repetitions as you can in a single breath: P-huh/P-huh/P-huh/P-huh/P-huh/P-huh.
2. Take another a deep breath in and do as many repetitions as you can in a single breath: P-huh/P-huh/P-huh/P-huh/P-huh/P-huh.
3. Take a third deep breath in and do as many repetitions as you can in a single breath: P-huh/P-huh/P-huh/P-huh/P-huh/P-huh.
4. Relax your breathing for 1 minute, then give me 3 explosive P-*huhs* with a breath between each: deep breath in, hold, and **P**-*huh*, deep breath in, hold, and **P**-*huh*, deep breath in, hold, and **P**-*huh*.
5. Take a deep breath, hold it for 2–3 seconds, and perform a controlled cough.

Some patients report that whenever they have a coughing spell or cannot clear, they just do a few explosive **P**–*huh* sounds and are able to clear.

Here is the take-home message: some techniques or devices may work exactly like the manufacturer's instructions describe or like your therapist taught you. Others may not help that much. Practice with different options to determine what works best for your body and lifestyle. Some people must mix and match using a different device in the morning compared to at night or when they are sick.

Unfortunately, unlike in a shoe store, we cannot try on different sizes and colors or take a walk around the store to see how they fit. These devices (even the cheapest ones) are costly, so pick an option and try it for a while. Work with your healthcare professional to see how to make it work better for you. Sometimes, you may need to try a different device. Gauge your improvement not just by how much mucus you expel, but also by how you feel in general and in terms of your ease of breathing.

I personally tell my patients that you need to think of yourselves like a professional athlete, musician, or singer. It is your time to train to be the best you can possibly be and although working on your respiratory health can be hard, you must work diligently for any of these tools to produce a positive outcome.

Chapter 17:

Lung Transplantation by René Hakkenberg

At some point, many Idiopathic Pulmonary Fibrosis (IPF) patients will consider getting a lung transplant. As we all know, there are currently no therapies to *cure* pulmonary fibrosis, and the medications presently available can at best, halt or slow the progression of the disease. They do not reverse fibrosis. But imagine if we could have a new set of lungs. Imagine a chance to start over and be free from this dreadful disease, from the constant shortness of breath (SOB), to be able to breathe again and ready to conquer the world again? The very idea sounds too wonderful to be true.

My name is René and in late 2017, when I was 75 years old, I was diagnosed with mild IPF. Over the next three years my condition continued to worsen, especially my shortness of breath. So, I decided to explore the option of getting a lung transplant. I contacted four well-known lung transplant centers and as requested, sent each of them my personal medical records including medications, surgeries, CT scans, and any other pertinent medical information. Once each confirmed receipt of my medical records, interviews were scheduled.

With each center I had at least a one-hour Zoom interview with the surgical team and/or the actual thoracic surgeon, during which we discussed the pros and cons of the surgery. In all four interviews, it became clear that my relatively advanced age could be a limiting factor – and for that reason, two of them rejected me.

Decision-makers at one center recommended against the transplant but were willing to proceed with the evaluation. Only one out of the four centers invited me to the complete their evaluation.

Several factors eventually made me decide against proceeding with the transplant. These included a higher mortality rate (age is the most significant risk factor for lung transplant survival), a more difficult and lengthy recovery, and the knowledge that my immune system would be suppressed by the anti-rejection drugs. This, in turn, would increase the risk of recurring skin cancer and/or other types of lung diseases. Another factor that weighed in my decision not to proceed was that my home is in the Dutch Caribbean Island of Bonaire, and I would have been required to travel from there to the US hospital many times. All in all, a lung transplant just did not seem like a viable option for me. But for you, it might be a completely different story – so please keep reading.

Your IPF Diagnosis

Idiopathic pulmonary fibrosis is a long-term disease in which scars develop on the lungs. This causes lung tissue to thicken, become stiff, and lose the elasticity of healthy lung tissue, which makes it hard for the patient to breathe. In fact, one of the first warning signs for someone with IPF is shortness of breath (SOB).

Initially, shortness of breath may be attributed to being out of shape, overweight, or simply getting older. Those who are physically fit may notice excessive SOB after exercising strenuously and may assume they have pushed themselves too hard. But over time, if we notice that the SOB has gotten worse, and walking up a staircase or up hilly terrain becomes difficult or impossible without stopping to rest, we instinctively know that something serious is going on and can no longer ignore the symptoms or chalk it up to "getting old." We eventually visit our family doctor, are referred to a pulmonologist, and are diagnosed with idiopathic pulmonary fibrosis – unwelcome news indeed.

Once the initial shock of the diagnosis wears off, it's natural for the patient to start rattling off questions for the doctor, such as, "well, what can you do for me? How can we treat this? What's our next step?" And there is nothing more frustrating and alarming than hearing the pulmonologist say: "There is no cure for IPF. I can prescribe medications, and they may help with your symptoms … but at best, they will slow the progression of the disease. Medications will not reverse the scarring in your lungs, and they may not stop the disease from getting worse."

As if that bombshell wasn't bad enough, you also learn that some patients have unbearable side effects from the medications. These may include nausea, vomiting, diarrhea, acid reflux, fatigue, loss of appetite, headache, dizziness, and skin problems. It isn't uncommon for IPF patients who experience some or all these side effects to stop using their medications. Quality of life becomes a major factor in such decisions.

So, you learned that you have IPF. You learned that there is no cure. You learned that you're going to get worse, even if you take medications because all they can do is slow down the scarring in your lungs. At this point, the pulmonologist may present you with the option of a lung transplant.

Exploring the Option of Lung Transplantation

Organ transplants can absolutely be considered marvels of modern medicine. They give people a new lease on life who might otherwise have no hope at all – yet these extraordinary lifesaving surgical techniques did not exist until the mid-twentieth century.

A Brief History

According to the United Network for Organ Sharing (UNOS), the first human organ transplant, took place in 1954. Twenty-three-year-old Richard Herrick was dying of kidney disease and was told there was nothing anyone could do for him. A young Harvard Medical School professor and surgeon named Dr. Joseph Murray did not agree with that. He believed it was possible to transplant a kidney from a healthy donor into the body of someone who needed it.

Called a "fool" for his belief in the possibilities of organ transplants, Dr. Murray took a healthy kidney from Herrick's twin brother and transplanted it into Herrick, saving the young man's life in the process. By the 1960s, liver, heart, and pancreas transplants were successfully being performed on a regular basis.

The first successful lung transplant was performed in 1971 by Dr. Fritz Derom in Belgium. The patient, a man in his twenties who worked as a sandblaster, had developed a type of pulmonary fibrosis known as end-stage silicosis. After the lung transplant, the man lived for 10 1/2 months – which was profound compared with previous attempts that resulted in patients surviving less than a month. By 1983, 40 successful lung transplants had been performed, and this number continued to increase over the following decades. Today, an estimated 2,000 lung transplants are performed in the United States each year.

A Serious Decision

It is important to talk to your doctor about the possibility of a transplant – and if your doctor doesn't mention it, don't hesitate to bring it up yourself. A lung transplant is a major and highly complex medical procedure, so it's essential for you to be well informed about every aspect of the surgery. It is not without risk, and recuperation can be difficult and slow.

Another important consideration is finances. A lung transplant, along with the necessary after-care, is *very* expensive, so make sure you know what your insurance provider will and won't pay for so that you are aware of all costs involved and can make sure you have your finances are in order. Also, besides the procedure itself, there will be major pre- and post-operational costs.

Before making your final decision about a transplant, ask yourself this question: will the risk of having a transplant exceed the expected benefits and life expectancy post-transplant – and answer the question truthfully. In other words, weigh your expected quality of life both with and without the operation. Make every effort to explore all aspects of the procedure and the process so you can make the best possible decision – for you.

Arm Yourself with Information

Once you've done your homework, found everything you could about lung transplants, read so much material that your eyes have started to cross, have weighed the pros and cons, understand the risks, and are ready to go ahead with the surgery ... what now? The first thing to know is that the window during which a transplant can take place is crucial. While the actual transplant is designed to address late-stage lung disease, early hospital selection and evaluation is important, so all preliminary testing is done when the patient is still relatively healthy.

Start by gathering information about lung transplant centers. An excellent source is the Scientific Registry of Transplant Recipients website (www.srtr.org), which provides a wealth of information about US transplant centers, including location, program overview, transplant rates, time to transplant, transplant outcomes, and a great deal more. Other countries may have similar websites.

You'll find contact information and links to each of the transplant centers so you can read about those of your choosing. Besides distance from home, you may want to consult with several lung transplant centers to determine which one suits you best and where you feel most comfortable, considering the proficiency of the medical staff, survival rates and other factors that are most important to you.

As mentioned, one extremely important consideration when choosing a transplant center is location. A lung transplant and recuperation will be a long process with numerous hospital visits, so the center's proximity to home is an important consideration. Keep in mind that once you are on the transplant list, *you must be able to be at the hospital within a very specific amount of time when called*, depending on the hospital. And you may get "the Call" at any time of the day or night, so you and your caregiver must be ready to leave at a moment's notice. Also, your transplant team will be your lifelong partner for post-operative follow up, making the distance from your home an even more important factor.

What to Consider Before Your Transplant

To be listed on the hospital's transplant list and qualify for the surgery, your disease stage must be relatively advanced. This is because the demand for healthy lungs far surpasses the supply. So those who need it most will tend to get preference (although this often varies from hospital to hospital).

Most hospitals will not perform transplants on a patient who is over 70 years old. Some, however, will go up to age 80 depending on the patient's physical and mental condition. Remember that if a transplant center rejects you can try another one or two more (as was my experience). Different hospitals have different requirements, so if one rejects you as a patient, another may not.

The hospital will request copies of all your medical information and history of previous operations or health problems, pulmonary function tests (PFTs), and six-minute walk tests. Other information gathered will include your age, height and weight, blood analyses, x-rays and high-resolution CT scans of your thorax, history of IPF diagnosis, biopsies, use of oxygen and oxygen saturation (at rest and when exercising), your exercise program and tolerance, current medications, your physical and mental condition, and lifestyle, and who your caregivers will be.

After all of these (and possibly other) criteria are reviewed and you're deemed a good candidate, the hospital will set a date for you to be evaluated at the transplant center.

What to Expect as a Transplant Candidate

As a candidate for a lung transplant, you will go through two to three weeks of testing at the transplant center. This will likely include physical, cognitive, and psychological testing. Financial matters will be discussed. Once all the tests are completed and have been evaluated by a team of specialists, you will meet with the transplant team. At that time, you will be given their best estimate of the risks of the operation and expected improvement of your functional status. The team will only list you as a patient if they believe that the benefits will outweigh the risks.

Keep in mind that it's not only the medical team that will make the decision to list you for the operation. *You* have a choice and ultimately, it will be you to decide whether to move forward with the procedure. So, it is of prime importance that you, supported by your caregiver(s), have a clear understanding of all the information you need to make a well-informed decision. Some patients consider the operation and all that it entails to be too overwhelming and decide against it.

Being "on the transplant list" or "listed," means that the transplant center has completed the evaluation and you have been approved for the procedure. Now you must await a donor for a unilateral (single) or bilateral (double) transplant. It is usually the medical team that will decide whether you should have one or two new lungs, depending on the benefits and risks of each option. Your medical history, age, availability of donor lungs, and the higher risk of transplanting two lungs compared with one, will all be taken into consideration. Be aware that a donor lung must be roughly the same size as your present lungs, so they fit in the chest cavity. You'll be informed of and have the right to decline if a donor is considered high risk (HIV-positive, drug user, etc.)

Whenever a lung becomes available in the U.S., the UNOS Organ Center will do computer matching. This, in turn, generates a list of potential recipients based on several factors, including blood type, medical urgency, lung size, and time on the waiting list.

You will need at least one caregiver, but most hospitals insist on two or more. As often as possible, your caregiver accompanies you during hospital visits before and after the transplant, during the evaluation, and throughout the period of recovery. The caregiver will be trained in normal patient care like medications and other situations, as well as what to do in case of an emergency. Considering the extremely important and expanded role a caregiver of a transplant patient will have both pre- and post-surgery, a spouse, family member or close friend are preferable caregivers. (See Chapter One on caregiving and the additional demands on a caregiver of a transplant patient.)

The expected period for the transplant operation and initial aftercare is typically from one to three weeks in the hospital, but could also be significantly longer, depending on any number of factors. Ask when it is likely that you'll get back on your feet, and have your medical team explain all the post-transplant medicines needed such as anti-rejection medications, antiviral drugs, and blood pressure drugs. Make sure you fully understand how the anti-rejection drugs work, their possible side-effects, and the dangers of postoperative complications. Because this plethora of drugs may negatively affect the working of healthy organs such as the kidneys and liver, you will be strongly advised to avoid using alcohol. Lungs are big organs and are exposed to air from the surroundings, so extreme care must be given to avoid any possible exposure to infections. This involves staying away from crowds or anyone with the flu or other medical problems.

Also, be aware of the need for continued and frequent testing post-transplant, probably starting with twice weekly with the frequency slowly being reduced, depending on your progress.

The Surgery

When "The Call" is received, you'll need to refrain from eating or drinking anything and accompanied by your caregiver, must leave for the hospital immediately. Upon your arrival, more last-minute tests will be done such an X-rays, blood analysis, and EKG. You must sign a consent form and possibly insurance papers and will be taken to the operating room. The anesthesiologist will put you to sleep so you will not feel any pain during the operation. A single lung transplant will usually take from four to six hours, while a double lung transplant will take up to ten hours. The exact time, of course, will vary from patient to patient.

Following your surgery, you will be taken to the intensive care unit and put on a ventilator to help you breathe. You'll usually remain on the ventilator for 24 to 48 hours, although for some patients it may be longer. You will be given immunosuppressant medications to prevent rejection of the lung(s), and antimicrobial medication to protect against lung infections.

After Your Lung Transplant

Even when your surgery is declared a shining success, life after the transplant will have its challenges. To reduce the risk of complications, you must follow the hospital care team's recommendations carefully, many of which will be lifelong.

Your body will perceive the new lung as a foreign object, and your immune system will naturally try to reject it. To prevent this from happening, you will need to take anti-rejection medications for the rest of your life. These are immune-suppressing medications that often carry side effects, and your transplant team will decide on the lowest but still effective dosage. Over time, as your recovery progresses, the dosage may be adjusted.

Despite these anti-rejection medications, about one-third of all transplant patients will suffer from acute cellular rejection (ACR), which usually happens between six months and a year after the transplant. Because ACR is asymptomatic, your transplant center will monitor you regularly for acute rejection; if you are diagnosed with ACR, your medical team will prescribe stronger anti-rejection medications. Depending on the hospital, this will mean a visit to the outpatient clinic once a week for up to several months to ensure your lung function keeps on improving.

While still in the hospital your transplant team will start a program of breathing and secretion clearance exercises and at some point, a pulmonary rehabilitation program, which should be continued after you are home.

Because the incision needs time to heal, you'll need to avoid excessive arm motion. Your rehabilitation program will be structured to avoid straining the incision. Also, it is generally recommended not to drive a car or lift more than 5 pounds for several months. If you notice any potential problems such as pain, swelling. redness, heat, leaking fluid, or fever, be sure to inform your care team immediately.

During these hospital visits you will be given some of the same tests you underwent before the operation, such as blood tests, PFTs, EKG, and possibly others. Over time, as your lung function improves, hospital visits will become less frequent.

After the transplant you will most likely enjoy a much better quality of life with easy breathing and *without* supplemental oxygen. Shortness of breath will hopefully be a thing of the past.

At all times, please be both grateful and mindful of the fact that another human being has lost his or her life for you to receive this precious and priceless gift. At some point, you may consider getting in touch with the deceased's family, if known, to express your appreciation. There have been many heartfelt stories of these sorts of meetings, and they often mean a great deal to all parties involved.

Final Thoughts

Going through a lung transplant and everything it entails is a major challenge – to put it mildly. You will be poked, prodded, and jabbed. It can be painful, frustrating, and stressful at times. You may even wonder if you made the right decision. Always remember, though, that most transplant patients are extremely pleased and relieved to have gone through the operation and would do it all over again.

For most patients, no longer having to live with constant shortness of breath, or needing to be plugged in to an oxygen tank, more than makes up for the difficulties of getting to that place.

As for me, René, I said early in this chapter that I had opted not to get the lung transplant. In the months and years after that, especially when I had severe IPF exacerbations and my condition worsened, I began to doubt whether I had made the right decision; I found myself wondering if I should have gone ahead with the surgery. These kinds of doubts are normal, of course. One can never be sure about the possible outcome of a lung transplant, whether it's a good option or whether it's not. And the conclusion I have arrived at is that I made the correct decision for me.

If you're reading this and are facing the same decision, remember that the only one who can make that decision for you is *you*.

Chapter 18:

Advance Planning for Your Legacy by Ronald Reid and Ann Kelley

If you have one of the interstitial lung diseases (ILDs), you may tend to think you have a defined timeline for your life, especially when you are newly diagnosed. All too often we think we are going to die soon; somewhere in that infamous 3–5-year prognosis quoted for IPF patients. But with better medicines and exercises, that prediction of survival has changed dramatically. No one has a definitive timeline, even though we know none of us live forever. For example, people in their 20s or 30s have caught Covid-19 and died young. Car crashes or cancer have no respect for age. The ways we might die are infinitely varied; but like taxes, death is one of the certainties of life.

My name is Ron, and I have been fortunate to live an interesting and fulfilling life. Four years ago, at the age of 68, I was diagnosed with IPF. After trying and then abandoning both Ofev and Esbriet, my plan now is to let nature take its course. I have a loving wife and two grown boys, so family is very much on my mind. My partner in writing the early stages of this chapter was Ann, who unfortunately succumbed to IPF before it was completed; more about her later.

Lung diseases give you the time and opportunity to sort through your preferences and arrangements about your eventual death. One of the best things you can give your children and the rest of your loved ones is the ability to talk about matters relating to your death. These are topics that many individuals and families, including my own children, seem to have difficulty discussing; many people are uncomfortable, or even downright squeamish, speaking about death. Usually, you will have to open the door to talking about it; lightening the mood by reminding them that "none of us get out of here alive" can help.

The best time to talk about these issues is now; proactively and before problems arise and sudden decisions must be made. Most of the suggestions in this chapter could apply to anyone in their senior years, not just those with ILD.

Why is this so important?

First, planning ahead ensures that your final wishes are honored. Do you want a big funeral or a small family gathering to celebrate your life? How do you want your remains to be handled? Who has authority to speak for you if you are no longer able? Don't leave your family guessing; let them know what you want to happen.

Most of us take great comfort in knowing those plans are in place and that we have set up arrangements as much as possible. As you will learn throughout this chapter, dying is not a simple business these days. The more various questions and uncertainties can be resolved, the less anxiety you are likely to feel as your end approaches.

Addressing these questions in advance is a wonderful gift to family or loved ones. You have removed the burden of them having to guess what you would prefer, and you set up a clear passage from this world to the next.

Dealing with the Legalities

Whether you are prince or pauper, several legal documents need to be in place to smooth your transition. Without them, the process will almost certainly be chaotic, expensive, and stressful for all involved. Three basic documents will cover most circumstances:

- Your Will
- Advance Directive for Health Care
- Durable Power of Attorney for Financial Affairs

To begin, do you have a legal Will in place? If so, well done! According to TD MoneyTalks, over half of Canadian adults don't have a signed Will; I don't think Americans are much different.

Unless your Will has been completed recently, you should have a fresh look to make sure that it fits with present circumstances and reflects your wishes. If necessary, update it with a lawyer (often an Elder Attorney who specializes in this area of law). For example, if you have divorced or changed your mind about where you want your money to go, a new Will is essential. The advice of a Financial Planner or a Certified Care Planner may also be useful in drawing up a Will that both respects your wishes and minimizes the tax burden associated with your death.

One aspect which is especially important is the appointment of your Executor (sometimes called Trustee). This person has the responsibility to ensure that all the steps necessary are carried out after your death and your wishes on disbursement of any assets are carried out as you directed. Your Executor must be someone you trust - a relative or a friend whom you know will be faithful to your wishes. They won't need to do all the detailed work themselves; your Executor usually will hire a lawyer (often the one who drew up the Will for you), as well as an accountant if your estate is complex.

When my wife and I recently reviewed our Wills, one helpful suggestion made by our lawyer was to draw up a separate list of keepsakes or other physical items that we want to leave to particular individuals. This helps keep the Will shorter and cleaner and makes it easier if we change our minds or want to add items. But please remember to destroy old copies of this list if you change your mind or make changes/updates. When an elderly maiden aunt of my mother passed away, her Executors found no fewer than three conflicting lists of where she wanted her furniture to go, creating all kinds of confusion in clearing out her house.

Next in line, and equally important, is to create an Advance Directive for your health care. This document lays out your wishes if you become incapacitated and cannot speak for yourself. For example, it may specify Do Not Resuscitate (DNR) orders under certain circumstances, or a wide range of other medical treatment instructions. In some jurisdictions, these documents are known as Living Wills or other terms. Advance Directives are intended to provide your medical team and your family with a clear expression of your wishes.

You can have your lawyer draft this document for you or download templates from the internet; usually two witnesses are required when you sign. Make sure you share your Advance Directive with your family doctor and your pulmonologist, as well as with the person or persons given the authority to carry out your Advance Directive. A family meeting may also be prudent so that all family members hear your wishes directly from you.

As part of your Advance Directive, you must appoint someone close to you as your Personal Care Power of Attorney for health care (wording for this person varies among jurisdictions; often referred to as the Attorney, which is confusing because they usually have no legal training). This is the person or persons who have the legal authority to make decisions on your behalf when you are no longer able. In most cases, this would simply involve ensuring that the terms of your Advance Directive are carried out. But some-times other circumstances arise that were not foreseen, and your Personal Care Attorney will have to make difficult decisions on your behalf in conjunction with the medical team. Almost always it is wise to have your lawyer draft this appointment for you so that there is no question about its authority.

One item you might consider including in your Advance Directive is organ donation if that is your wish. It is important for your healthcare team to be informed about the potential for organ donation in advance. While your lungs obviously won't be of much interest except perhaps as a research resource, a surprisingly wide range of other organs could save or improve someone's life if you chose to donate, despite having IPF.

Even if your life and assets seem very simple, it is also important for you to appoint a "Durable Power of Attorney" for your financial affairs. This person takes over when you become unable to make financial decisions yourself and has authority until your death. Their responsibility could stretch all the way from running your business to just making sure the rent, mortgage and other bills are paid while you are still alive, depending on what powers you have assigned to this person. You will want legal help in drafting this document, because it entrusts a lot of power to the person named as your Durable Power of Attorney for financial affairs. Keep in mind that you will likely be unaware of how they are spending your money, so it needs to be someone you fully trust. If you have any doubts, talk to your lawyer about how to limit their powers, or choose someone else.

In some cases, the same person can serve as your Power of Attorney for both healthcare and financial affairs. Depending on your circumstances, the person acting as your Durable Power of Attorney may also carry-on being Executor of your Will. Note that regulations affecting these powers vary from state to state in the U.S., as well as in Canada and other countries. In most cases, it is prudent to have your lawyer draft the documents for both the Personal Care Power of Attorney and the Durable Power of Attorney for financial affairs. This can be done at the same time as you review your Will.

Don't forget to talk to your potential Power of Attorney agents in advance to make sure they are willing! You should also go over the relevant documents with them, so there are no surprises when they are called on to act.

Getting things organized

You can make life immeasurably easier for your Executor and your family by providing a list of documents and contacts for their use after your death. Our lawyer provided a very helpful template to fill in this information; you may also be able to find something similar on the internet. Some of that information includes:

- Contacts to notify family, list of friends, business colleagues if appropriate, doctors, lawyer, insurance contacts, oxygen provider, etc.; if possible, add a list of contact information for friends and family.
- Funeral home (make arrangements in advance) and burial or cremation arrangements.
- Obituary: some people write their own; others leave it to family.
- Bank accounts (make one a joint account with your Durable Power of Attorney to allow them access, and with your Executor since most accounts in your name alone are frozen upon your death).
- Retirement plans and insurance plans; this is also a good time to check to ensure that the correct people are listed as

beneficiaries for each plan and that the policies are noted as payable on death.

- Safety deposit box, including where the key is located; or have the bank list your Executor as a co-holder of the box.
- Copies of any other legal documents and associated directives.
- Passwords for your computer and programs your heirs may wish to access.

Place this information or documents in a file that is easily accessed when needed, and make sure your Executor or other close family members know where they are located. If needed, your lawyer will have copies of your Will and other legal documents on file. Some of these contacts such as banks and insurance companies will require a copy of your death certificate, but that is one task you can't plan in advance!

While you are still able, another useful task is to plan your own funeral or celebration of life, as well as the disposition of your remains. This starts with choosing a funeral home; ask your family and friends for recommendations, and if you can, arrange to visit a few of these businesses in advance to find one that meets your needs. There are lots of decisions to be made, and each decision has a price tag, so setting up your plans in advance can have financial advantages. Oftentimes, making arrangements in advance and paying for these services beforehand will be significantly less expensive. Leaving all these decisions to your family to make during the shock of your passing can result in a much more costly service than you would have preferred.

Generally speaking, it is much better for you to make your own choices on such matters as:

- Cremation or embalming or some other treatment of your body. An increasing number of us are looking at "green burials," using a simple casket and no chemicals to allow our bodies to naturally degrade back into the earth; this option needs to be approved in advance to avoid difficulties.
- Provision of opportunities for "viewing," as well as a formal funeral service.
- Choice of cemetery or final resting place for your ashes, depending on the choices you have made above.
- Whether you prefer a fancy commercial casket or a plain pine box.
- An opportunity for family and friends to gather, either immediately after a traditional funeral or sometime later; the funeral home will be glad to provide this service (at a price), or your family can arrange some kind of celebration on their own.

Every person and every family will have their own preferences about how to honor your passing; if you have your own wishes, it is best to make those arrangements in advance.

Leaving a Legacy (*Adapted in part with permission from Kim Fredrickson to Noah Greenspan from her book, Pulmonary Fibrosis Journey, 2018*)

In its broadest sense, a legacy is something handed down from one generation to the next. All of us will pass on a legacy of some kind to our family, friends, and coworkers. The type of legacy depends on us. People often think this means leaving a financial inheritance. But it is much broader; your legacy could include financial blessings, meaningful memories, values, knowledge, and wisdom.

It's normal to want to be remembered and feel like we made a difference to the world in large or small ways. We want our lives to have mattered and to be a positive influence on generations to come. The legacy we leave is about far more than material things. Some of the great ideas that PF patients shared with Kim to create meaningful memories include:

- If you have any property with family significance, take photos and record its background, owner, and its family relationship.
- Make scrapbooks with old photos and mementos for your spouse, kids, grandchildren, and special friends; they will be cherished for years to come.
- Gather your favorite recipes and create a cookbook to leave to friends and loved ones.
- Write letters or journals to loved ones; think about everything you want to tell them and write it down for them to enjoy over and over. A great place to let your spouse or partner know how much you love them and how much you wish they will find happiness after you're gone.
- Let your kids and grandkids know how proud you are of them and how much you'll miss them. This might be a brief journal noting fun times you shared, ways you want to encourage them, and things you love about them.

- If you won't see a loved one attain a momentous life event such as graduation, marriage, birth of first child, etc., buy special gifts or write a letter to be given to them later.
- Make video or audio recordings, so that your loved ones can see you or hear your voice. For grandchildren, this might be a recording of you reading children's stories. For older children, it might be about your life growing up.

Some of these ideas might strike a chord with you, others not so much. Kim's book (*Pulmonary Fibrosis Journey; A Counselor and Fellow Patient Walks with You*) has other ideas on how to make memories that will be meaningful for those you leave behind.

If you can bless your family financially with individual gifts, this time-honored tradition is always warmly received. But there are other ways to leave a financial legacy as well. One way is to give to charities that reflect your heart and values. That might be through an educational institution to endow a scholarship for future students in an area that has special meaning for you. For my wife and I, our charity of choice is a local land trust that has done much to preserve special areas for wildlife. We chose to donate to them through a life insurance policy. For any charitable gifts, be sure to check with your tax and financial advisors for the best way to accomplish your charitable goals most effectively.

Another form of legacy is to share your values and life lessons. Some values and ethics come to mind easily, like honesty, love, generosity, kindness, gratitude, forgiveness, faith, and compassion. Other topics, such as what gives life meaning, keys to a happy marriage, and how to raise a happy and responsible kid, are more difficult. Sharing your own experience and encouraging your family to think about these questions can be a valuable legacy as well.

Sharing your knowledge and wisdom in ways that may benefit future generations can come in many forms, including but not limited to:

- Creating a video: this can be an effective way of communicating advice, heartfelt wisdom, and stories passed down through the generations, because your heirs will treasure hearing and seeing your message. Share what you have learned from difficult experiences, along with events and connections that have brought you joy. You might even talk about what you would do differently if you had the chance.
- Passing on health information about yourself and others in your family may be important for future generations to take advantage of advancements in science and DNA testing. This information can help prevent illnesses, guide preventative care, and aid in diagnosis. IPF is one example of an illness which in some patients appears to have a genetic link. In my case, after I was diagnosed, I discovered that an aunt and an uncle on my mother's side both had IPF late in their lives. Not close enough to establish a definitive genetic link, for now at least, but may be valuable information at some future date.
- Documenting your genealogy is a wonderful way to let your kids and grandkids understand where you and they came from. Besides using specialized websites for family history, you can add personal stories and anecdotes about family

members and your relationships. What a rich legacy to pass down to your loved ones!

One part of your legacy that you don't want to pass on is negative relationships. No doubt you, like me, have some messy relationships in your life. Ask yourself if there is someone in your life you would like to apologize to. You may have unresolved issues with family members and friends; it's almost impossible not to. Part of anyone's legacy might be doing what we can to resolve unfinished business or mend broken relationships before we die. Asking for forgiveness and forgiving yourself and others for mistakes made is freeing and will help give you peace.

Don't spend too much of your energy on fixing the past, however. The time we have with family and friends is precious to us and to them. Watch for opportunities to talk, play, and enjoy one another. Take a risk and go deeper to talk about important things. Listen deeply and watch for opportunities to encourage your loved ones. They long to receive your approval, attention, and love. These moments of love and connection will live on in their hearts.

This section on Leaving a Legacy has many suggestions and may seem a little overwhelming. You may not be at the point of being able to act on them, and that's OK. When you have time and energy, choose one or two that appeal to you, and start with them. If that brings you joy and satisfaction, choose another. Trust your heart, and only move forward with the ones that fit you and your life.

The End Stages of Pulmonary Fibrosis/ILD

Chances are you have fought hard against your lung disease. You have done everything possible to postpone your death. Perhaps you have gone through the difficult evaluation process for new lungs, but you have been turned down, or too much time has passed with no matching transplant in sight. At some point, you know in your heart that the end is coming for you.

What will your final days or weeks be like? If your battle against lung disease has left you bitter and disillusioned, you might envision them in the words of the Welsh poet Dylan Thomas:

> *"Do not go gentle into that good night,*
> *Old age should burn and rave at close of day;*
> *Rage, rage against the dying of the light."*

But for many of us, the idea of a "good death" has changed considerably from this angry screed. When I asked my family doctor about the dying process with IPF, he described it as a diminishing series of circles. Gradually your abilities diminish; over time you sleep more, and your social life diminishes too. As your lung's capacity to provide oxygen lessens, other organs begin to fail as well; at some point you appear to be asleep but fall into a coma; your breathing slows and becomes irregular; eventually it stops.

That gentle process is very much reflected in a 2020 book by Dr. Kathryn Mannix called *"With the End in Mind: Dying, Death, and Wisdom in an Age of Denial."* After observing thousands of deaths over the past 40 years, she has noted a similar pattern of dying in almost all gravely ill patients. (Note this does not include patients who have suffered accidents or other sudden events where the life-saving technology of emergency wards is being employed to attempt to defy death.)

Our friend Ann's death is such a fine example of this process, and her passing in April 2021 has become a valuable contribution to this chapter.

Ann was an Alabama grandmother who had been an active participant in our IPF learning sessions, video conferences and in the preparation and writing of this book. She and I volunteered to take on this final chapter, but part-way through, she sent me a message expressing her apologies that she was unable to participate further. She was in a hospice. It soon became clear that she knew her life was ending, and within a week we received news that it had. She died gently, surrounded by her family and as in control of the situation as she could be. In a gesture that was typical of Ann, she left her family a letter, telling them she loved them and was proud of them. She told them as well how proud she was to be part of our book-writing process.

Ann had planned her death well in advance and had made arrangements for hospice accommodation in her final days. She was at peace with her fate because she had strong religious beliefs and was at peace with her God. She died as she planned, in the cradle of her family and in the setting of her choice.

Choosing where you wish to die is not always feasible because emergency situations may get in the way of well-laid plans. However, you can make your preferences known, and discuss them with your close family, caregivers, and medical staff, and often those wishes can be followed.

- Many of us would prefer to die at home, in familiar surroundings. This may depend on whether family and at-home programs, including staff such as Personal Support Workers are available to help. The type of home is also vital - a single-story bungalow with easy access to bathrooms is much easier to manage than houses with stairs. Spending your last days at home likely also involves creating a "Home Crisis Plan" with input from your doctors and hospital emergency officials.

- Another choice may be at a hospice, which are increasingly available in local communities to provide care and comfort through your final days. Most of us think of hospice care as end-of life residential care, and indeed that is a central part of their role. But hospices often also provide care in your own home, which focuses on providing care that ensures your comfort and well-being, recognizing that further treatment aimed at recovery is futile. So, find out what hospice services are available in your community and talk to them well in advance.

- Dying at a hospital may not be your first choice, but this is the reality for many patients, especially if they have not signed an Advance Directive to decline medical procedures that will keep you alive longer.

No matter where you spend your final days, your care should be focused on making sure you are as comfortable as possible. Until the happy day when a cure is found for IPF and other ILDs, anything else would be pointless.

Palliative care is focused on improving the overall wellness and comfort of individuals in the late stages of serious illnesses. It addresses both the symptoms and the stress of living with a chronic illness. It also involves support for loved ones or care-givers. Palliative care can take place alongside other treatments intended to extend your life. In essence, palliative care is intended to address your individual needs, and to provide the resources to do so, whether physical, emotional, or spiritual.

When you think about how you would like your last year to unfurl, contacting a palliative care team can be an important part of those plans. They do much more than simply providing the appropriate drugs to temper any pain or distress you may be feeling. Their role may also address emotional or family issues and help you through planning for a graceful exit.

For IPF patients, the five primary symptoms that will likely occur during the end stages of your disease are shortness of breath, cough, fatigue, anxiety and depression, and fear of the unknown. Palliative care provides medicines or counseling to deal with each of these, in increased doses as needed. For example, supplementary oxygen may be provided at greater levels to provide comfort as your lungs weaken. Perhaps the greatest fear of IPF/ILD patients is a feeling of suffocation or drowning in their final moments; this too can be controlled by medications; Ann's peaceful death is the norm for those under palliative care.

Your doctor can refer you to a palliative care specialist, or you can search the resources of the website GetPalliativeCare.org to find services near you. Don't wait until your final days to access the palliative care specialists and facilities near you; make use of them as early and often as you can.

In some jurisdictions (including Canada, Netherlands, Switzerland, and some U.S. States), legal provisions for Medical Assistance in Dying allow a person to request the assistance of a doctor to end their life if certain criteria are met. Otherwise, assisting with a planned death is a criminal offence. For many patients, religious or ethical objections rule out this possibility, and for most IPF patients, good palliative care can make it unnecessary. However, if you wish to consider this option, discuss it with your medical team and loved ones.

Another of our IPF patient group, John, sent us this personal reminder about one final experience that can be shared with a patient and their family or friends:

"The deathbed vigil is very often a topic that's unspoken and extremely difficult for the family, but it is a time that will be important to your loved one as they depart. Your loved one needs to feel the warmth and love of their family and overall unity of the parties present is of the utmost importance. Share the old anecdotes, songs, jokes, reminiscing on past trips and happy times. This is a labor of love provided for the patient and a joyous moment for them as they

make their departure. This is a time for you to thank them for the experiences you gained knowing them and to reinforce that you will continue to love and appreciate them. A peaceful loving transition will ease their burden and hopefully bring you to terms with your feelings. I won't burden you with what a higher power might think; you must live within your own boundaries of spirituality. Please make this final slice of time one of love and joyous remembrance; this will surely be a precious legacy memory."

What John is suggesting is the opposite of denial; rather the full involvement of those who love you in your passing from this world. For those of us who have struggled so often to breathe, being surrounded by love as we take our last breath somehow seems fitting. May it be so for all and every one of us.

Final Thoughts & Motivations by Noah Greenspan, PT, DPT, CCS, EMT-B

"Whether you think you can or think you can't—you're right."
– Henry Ford

I often encounter people during some of the worst times of their lives. Perhaps they have been newly diagnosed or maybe they are experiencing an exacerbation or progression of their existing disease or some other setback in their lives. This can be difficult to cope with from both a physical and emotional perspective. After all, not being able to breathe can be incredibly stressful, anxiety provoking, *and* depressing.

Life with a chronic illness can (and will) have its ups and downs. But guess what. So can life *without* a chronic illness. Ups and downs are a natural part of being human. Regardless of who you are, some days will shine brighter than others and other days, things will get dark. Sometimes, everything in your life will seem perfect and sometimes, well, quite simply, they will suck. The key is not to get stuck in "Suckville."

"When we are no longer able to change a situation, we are challenged to change ourselves." – Victor Frankl

Please don't think that I am minimizing your situation. I am *not*. I also understand that what I am saying is easier said than done and sometimes, no matter what you do, it can be hard to dig yourself out of that hole. That's when it's time to ask for help, whether it be from your doctor or other health care professional, friends or family members, clergyman or clergywoman, dog, cat, bird; or whomever or whatever it may be that helps pick you up when you're down.

My work is often challenging in so many ways, which is one of the things I love about it. I often get to go back and forth between a physiology-based, science-intensive role, to a pop-psychology feel-good pick-me-upper, to a locker room halftime speech all in the same day. In the end, I decided to incorporate a little of each here, with the purpose of motivating you, giving you some helpful tips and sending you back out on the field, feeling ready to kick some butt.

I have also decided to share some of my favorite quotes with you; particularly those in which, I, myself find comfort or motivation or that otherwise inspire me when I am being faced with my own personal challenges, of which there have been many. Hopefully, you will find them helpful as well. If not, feel free to cross mine out and write in your own.

"The only constant in life is change." – Greek Philosopher, Heraclitus of Ephesus

The Greek philosopher, Heraclitus of Ephesus, lived from 535 BC-475 BC and is best known for his doctrine on change being central to the universe. This goes hand in hand with "this too, shall pass," attributed to either Persian Sufi poets or King Solomon of the bible depending on your source.

"This, too, shall pass." – Persian Sufi Poets or King Solomon

These quotes remind us that change is inevitable and that we should not find it surprising when things in our lives shift, be it for better or for worse. In fact, we should be more surprised when things stay the same. Another piece of advice to be gleaned from those messages is to try to embrace the change, roll with the punches, soak in life's beautiful moments and push through the challenges because *nothing* lasts forever; again, for better or for worse.

What Can We Do?

According to British philosopher, Alan Watts, "By replacing fear of the unknown with curiosity, we open ourselves up to an infinite stream of possibility. We can let fear rule our lives, or we can become childlike with curiosity, pushing our boundaries, leaping out of our comfort zones, and accepting what life puts before us." For our purposes, I take this quote to mean that we can't alleviate stress-related *symptoms* unless we address their underlying cause. Here are some ideas of ways to make your life easier, happier a.

Get Educated!

Fear of the unknown can very often worsen or intensify whatever situation you are dealing with. When it comes to finding out about your medical condition, everybody is different and has different levels of "wanting to know." For me, personally, it is almost always better to find out as much information as I can, and what I can do to deal with the problem head-on.

This can be especially important for people living with a chronic illness. By learning as much as you can about your disease, its associated symptom, and available treatments, you will be in a better position to make decisions regarding your care and your life. In addition, this understanding can help you gain a greater sense of control, reduce your day-to-day stress, and contribute to your overall sense of well-being.

"Knowledge is the antidote to fear." – **Ralph Waldo Emerson**

In an ideal world, your doctor or his staff would have all the time in the world to sit down with you and explain your diagnosis, test results, and treatment options. However, while many medical professionals make patient education a regular part of their practice, we know that others simply don't have the time to do this for each patient.

Thankfully, there are many other resources that can help you find the information you need. As I have mentioned from the start, there is *a lot* of information on the Internet. To be sure that the material you are finding is both relevant and accurate, I would suggest *starting* with some of the official disease-related foundations and associations. Of course, we are biased toward our own Pulmonary Wellness Foundation but we also like the American Lung Association and their Better Breathers Clubs, the Pulmonary Fibrosis Foundation, and the Pulmonary Hypertension Association, among others.

I would also like to invite you to view my *Ultimate Pulmonary Wellness* Webinars. During these 1-2-hour-plus webinars, I discuss key components of optimal disease management as well as having the honor of having many of the tippy-top specialists in their respective fields as my guests.

The Ultimate Pulmonary Wellness Webinar Series can be found online at:

www.PulmonaryWellness.com/Webinars

Get Support!

Humans are, by nature, social creatures and we know that social support plays a huge role in shaping our emotional health and enhancing our quality of life. Chronic harmful emotions like stress, anxiety and depression can feel exponentially more oppressive when we are dealing with them in isolation. We all have busy lives but spending time with loved ones can significantly improve your emotional state, mental health, and physical well-being.

While the support of family and friends is extremely important, this can sometimes present its own challenges. As an example, you may not feel comfortable sharing certain aspects of your disease with them. You may feel like they will not be able to understand your situation, or you may not want to burden them with your concerns.

This is where a support group can be a tremendous help. By belonging to a group in which, people have the same or similar condition, you will come to realize that you are *not* alone. You will have the opportunity to interact with people who are going through similar struggles, and who knows? You may even be able to serve as a resource to someone else in need. Whether in-person, by telephone, or online, support groups can help you learn from the experience of others and share your own in return.

The UPW Facebook Group can be found online at:

www.facebook.com/groups/UltimatePulmonaryWellness

Think Positive!

Optimism and/or pessimism can have a major impact on your physical, mental, and emotional health. I realize that maintaining a positive attitude is sometimes easier said than done, but people who have a positive attitude often have a greater ability to deal with stress. Taking steps to reframe your attitude and negative self-talk will prepare you to cope more effectively with stressful situations and to fight off anxiety and depression.

Take steps to surround yourself with positive influences. If you're constantly being assaulted by cynical people, negativity, or rude comments; or depressing or anxiety-provoking TV shows or other media outlets, you will have a much harder time breaking the cycle of negativity.

"The most important decision is to be in a good mood."
– Voltaire

LOL!

There's a reason why we often call laughter the best medicine. Laughter can lower our stress level, decrease anxiety, and reduce depression. Laughing can relieve both physical and emotional tension in our bodies, reducing the level of stress hormones in the blood and stimulating the release of endorphins, relieving pain, and promoting healthy immune function.

Finding a way to laugh productively in stressful or depressing circumstances may seem challenging at first, but, like anything, it gets easier with practice. Make humor an intentional part of your life. In the end, the method doesn't matter as much as trying to lighten the mood, whenever possible.

"We need more kindness, more compassion, more joy, and more laughter. I definitely want to contribute to that." – **Ellen DeGeneres**

Making the Change

Living with a chronic respiratory disease is not easy and can trigger negative emotions such as stress, anxiety, and depression, both in the moment and over the long-term. One of the ironies is that when we're feeling stressed, anxious, depressed, or angry, we often engage in the exact opposite behaviors that we should. We decrease our participation in healthy activities like exercise and increase our participation in unhealthy behaviors like eating poorly or using tobacco.

Again, please understand that I am not minimizing your feelings or saying that it will be easy. I recognize and appreciate the gigantic emotional toll that living with a chronic illness can have on a person's life, especially one in which shortness of breath is a primary symptom. The good news is that you *do* have the power to change and there *are* things that you can do to minimize your symptoms and improve your life.

"You're braver than you believe and stronger than you seem, and smarter than you think." – **Christopher Robin**

As far as any of us knows, we only get one life to live and I'm going to fight for it. I may go down, but if I'm going down, you'd better believe I'm going down fighting tooth and nail and for every breath. In the case of Ultimate Pulmonary Wellness, this means gathering up your army, and using every weapon and tool you have at your disposal. Your army includes your family, friends, doctors, and other healthcare professionals, among others. Your tools and weapons are your medications, exercising, eating well, managing your stress and anxiety, and taking steps to prevent infection.

For today, *try* not to focus on what you don't have or what you can't do. Focus on the things that you can do and *do them well.* If you can help someone else in the process, that's all the better. Answer someone's question, share your experience, express a few words of encouragement to someone that is struggling…and *breathe.* You are alive! Make sure you don't forget to live. I am with you. Make it a great one, my friends.

"Never, never, never, never give up!" – **Winston Churchill**

"Imperfection is beauty, madness is genius and it's better to be absolutely ridiculous than absolutely boring." - **Marilyn Monroe**

Index